# Pocket Picture Guides

# Diabetes
## Second Edition

GW00729202

**Pocket Picture Guides**

# Diabetes
## Second Edition

### H Jonathan Bodansky
MB, ChB (Hons), MD (Liverpool), MRCP

Consultant Physician
The General Infirmary at Leeds
Senior Clinical Lecturer
University of Leeds
West Yorkshire, UK.

**Ⅵ Wolfe**

ISBN 0 7234 2053 X

Printed in the UK
Produced by BPCC Hazell Books Ltd, Aylesbury, Bucks., UK
Set in Sabon and Frutiger

First Edition © Copyright 1989 by Gower Medical
Publishing.
Second Edition © Copyright 1994 by Times Mirror
International Publishers Limited.
Published in 1994 by Wolfe Publishing, an imprint of Times
Mirror International Publishers Limited.

For full details of all Times Mirror International Publishers Limited titles,
please write to Times Mirror International Publishers Limited, Lynton
House, 7–12 Tavistock Square, London WC1H 9LB, England.

# PREFACE

This Pocket Picture Guide hopes to provide a basic working knowledge about all aspects of diabetes mellitus in a concise pictorial form. I hope that it will be useful for nurses, medical students and doctors in learning about diabetes.

Since the publication of the first edition of this book, the diabetes control and complications trial (DCCT) in the USA has shown clearly that tighter control of blood glucose levels in patients with insulin-dependent diabetes (IDDM) may help to prevent the appearance or progression of the chronic complications of diabetes. Further understanding of the cause of IDDM has been gained by the finding that glutamic acid decarboxylase (GAD) may be one of the pancreatic islet cell antigens against which islet cell antibodies are directed. The biochemical basis of non-insulin-dependent diabetes (NIDDM) is under intensive scrutiny using molecular biology techniques and further understanding about its cause is strongly anticipated.

I am grateful to my teachers in diabetes, the late Professor Andrew Cudworth, Dr John Wales and Dr David Barnett and to the many colleagues and patients from whom I have learnt so much. Invaluable help has been provided by the publishers. Without the assistance, advice and encouragement of my wife, Valerie, this book and my personal development would have been impossible.

HJB
Leeds

# ACKNOWLEDGEMENTS

The author would like to thank the following individuals for providing illustrative material:

Dr SGR Aparicio, Leeds (Fig. 101); Dr D Barnett, Leeds (Figs 22, 26, 45, 73, 75, 78, 80–83, 116, 120, 121, 123–125, 128, 143, 145, 147, 148, 151, 152, 154); Professor G-F Bottazzo, London (Figs 16 & 17); Professor KD Buchanan, Belfast (Fig. 14); Dr JMH Buckler, Leeds (Figs 156–158); Dr PM Chennells, Leeds (Fig. 76); the late Professor AG Cudworth, London (Figs 79, 115, 141, 149 & 150); Dr T Donini, Minimed, Neuilly sur Seine (Fig. 46); the late Dr MI Drury, Dublin (Fig. 163); Dr ME Edmonds, London (Figs 119 & 122); Dr A Foulis, Glasgow (Fig. 23); Professor EM Gale, London (Fig. 60); the late Professor W Gepts, Brussels (Fig. 15); the late Professor W Gepts and Dr PA in't Veld, Brussels (Fig. 21); Dr P Gibson, Leeds (Fig. 77); Dr M Goodfield, Leeds (Figs 134–136, 138, 139, 142, 144); Mr J Hillman, Leeds (Figs 85, 86, 89, 91–96); the late Dr JT Ireland, Glasgow (Figs 102 & 103); Professor DJA Jenkins, Toronto (Fig. 37c); Dr RH Jones, London (Fig. 20); Mr B Martin, Leeds (Figs 87 & 98); Mr T Metcalfe, Leeds (Fig. 90); Dr DWM Pearson and Professor JM Stowers, Aberdeen (Fig. 36); Dr R Pujol-Borell and Professor G-F Bottazzo, London (Fig. 18); Dr P Silverton, Leeds (Fig. 22); Mr DJ Spalton, Leeds (Figs 88 & 97); Professor RB Tattersall, Nottingham (Figs 50, 52 & 53); Dr JK Wales, Leeds (Figs 24, 25 & 153); Professor JD Ward, Sheffield (Figs 114, 118, 130, 131); Dr PJ Watkins, London (Figs 106, 129 & 146); Dr MA Waugh, Leeds (Figs 137 & 140); Mr RAF Whitelocke, London (Fig. 99); Dr PG Wiles, Manchester (Fig. 133); Dr EJ Will, Leeds (Figs 109 & 110); Professor P Zimmet, Melbourne (Fig. 7).

# CONTENTS

# DEFINITIONS, CLASSIFICATION AND AETIOLOGY

Diabetes mellitus is a syndrome characterized by chronic hyperglycaemia. A high blood glucose level produces an osmotic diuresis, leading to the typical symptoms of polyuria, nocturia, thirst, weakness and weight loss. The World Health Organization (WHO) provides blood glucose values for the diagnosis of diabetes in the fasting state and two hours after a glucose load in a standardized oral glucose tolerance test (OGTT). In most cases, it is unnecessary to perform an OGTT as the diagnosis of diabetes is readily confirmed by a high random blood glucose value and typical symptoms. However, an OGTT may confirm, or refute, the diagnosis of diabetes in borderline cases. To help classify these borderline cases, the WHO introduced the concept of 'impaired glucose tolerance' (IGT). Subjects with IGT do not have frank diabetes but may progress to it.

| GLUCOSE VALUES FOR DIABETES | | | |
|---|---|---|---|
| **Random sample (mmol/l)** | | | |
| | diabetes likely | diabetes uncertain | diabetes unlikely |
| venous plasma | ≥11.1 | 5.5–<11.1 | <5.5 |
| venous blood | ≥10.0 | 4.4–<10.0 | <4.4 |
| capillary plasma | ≥12.2 | 5.5–<12.2 | <5.5 |
| capillary blood | ≥11.1 | 4.4–<11.1 | <4.4 |
| **Standardized OGTT (mmol/l)** | | | |
| | | diabetes | IGT |
| venous Plasma | fasting | ≥ 7.8 | < 7.8 |
| | 2h | ≥11.1 | 7.8–<11.1 |
| venous blood | fasting | ≥ 6.7 | < 6.7 |
| | 2h | ≥10.0 | 6.7–<10.0 |
| capillary plasma | fasting | ≥ 7.8 | < 7.8 |
| | 2h | ≥12.2 | 8.9–<12.2 |
| capillary blood | fasting | ≥ 6.7 | < 6.7 |
| | 2h | ≥11.1 | 7.8–<11.1 |

**Fig. 1** WHO criteria for diagnosis of diabetes mellitus. Criteria are provided for diagnosis from samples taken at random, after a fast or following an OGTT. A load of 75g glucose is currently used in the OGTT as a compromise between 100g in the USA and 50g in Europe. The diagnostic criteria vary depending on whether the sample is whole blood or plasma, venous or capillary. The OGTT should be performed in the morning after an overnight fast and the subject should not be on a carbohydrate-restricted diet, but should be eating his or her usual diet.

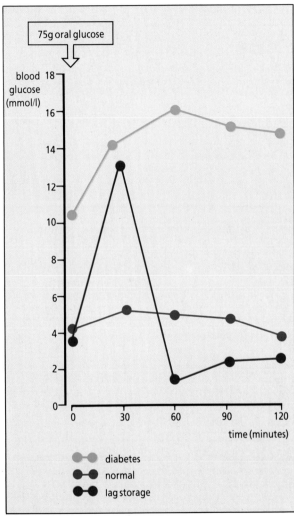

**Fig. 2** Typical curves during a 75g OGTT. Patients with previous upper gastrointestinal tract surgery (e.g. gastrectomy or gastroenterostomy) may demonstrate early hyperglycaemia followed by hypoglycaemia ('lag storage' or 'steeple curve'). This is due to rapid absorption of glucose followed by acute insulin secretion and does not constitute diabetes. A low renal threshold for glucose may cause glycosuria without diabetes or IGT.

## CLASSIFICATION OF DIABETES MELLITUS

insulin-dependent (IDDM)

non-insulin-dependent (NIDDM) (a) obese
(b) non-obese

secondary to pancreatic disease, e.g. chronic pancreatitis,
haemochromatosis and pancreatectomy

malnutrition-related (MRDM)

secondary to endocrine disease, e.g. Cushing's syndrome,
acromegaly and phaeochromocytoma

drug-induced, e.g. steroids and thiazides

associated with genetic syndromes, e.g. Friedreich's ataxia and
dystrophia myotonica

impaired glucose tolerance (IGT)

gestational diabetes

**Fig. 3** Modified classification of diabetes mellitus from that devised by the National Diabetes Data Group. In the Western World, most cases of diabetes are non-insulin-dependent and only a minority are insulin-dependent. In developing countries, diabetes may be associated with a degree of malnutrition and chronic pancreatic damage in which protein restriction and toxicity from cassava may be involved. Occasionally, cases are drug-induced, secondary to pancreatic or endocrine disease or associated with various rare genetic syndromes.

| IDDM | NIDDM |
|---|---|
| ketosis prone | non-ketosis prone |
| insulin treatment mandatory | insulin treatment optional |
| onset often acute | insidious onset |
| usually non-obese | obese or non-obese |
| typical onset in youth but any age possible | onset usually over 50 years of age but maturity-onset diabetes of youth is a variant |
| HLA-DR3 and DR4 common | HLA unrelated |
| islet cell antibodies | no islet cell antibodies |
| family history positive in 10% of cases | family history positive in 30% of cases |
| 30 – 50% concordance in identical twins | nearly 100% concordance in identical twins |

**Fig. 4** Characteristic features of IDDM and NIDDM. On clinical grounds, patients can be divided into insulin-dependent and non-insulin-dependent, although not all subjects are easy to classify. This is because any diabetic patient can be treated with insulin, but not all insulin-treated patients are insulin-dependent. A history of ketoacidosis or ketonuria under conditions of metabolic stress provides evidence of insulin-dependence. The concept of Type I and Type II diabetes not only encompasses clinical aspects, but also includes aetiological and pathological mechanisms. The two syndromes form indistinct entities and are not strictly synonymous with IDDM and NIDDM. Type I/IDDM and Type II/NIDDM each have certain characteristic features. However, no feature absolutely distinguishes one type from the other.

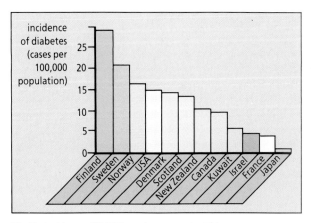

**Fig. 5** Incidence of IDDM in various countries. This seems most frequent in northern Europe or in populations derived from there, being commoner with increasing latitude. This may imply a genetic predisposition in northern European populations or may be the effect of local environmental agents.

| PREVALENCE OF NIDDM IN VARIOUS POPULATIONS | | |
| --- | --- | --- |
| country | ethnic group | prevalence (%) |
| Australia | Caucasian | 3.4 |
| USA | general | 6.8 |
| | Caucasian | 6.4 |
| | Negroid | 9.9 |
| | Mexican American | 10.6 |
| | Pima Indians | 34.1 |
| Nauru | Micronesian | 30.3 |
| Fiji | Melanesian | 6.9 |
| | Indian | 14.8 |
| Western Samoa | Polynesian | 4.9 |
| Papua New Guinea | Melanesian | 0.0 |

**Fig. 6** Prevalence of NIDDM in various populations. This appears to occur world-wide and is often related, although not necessarily, to increasing body weight. Certain inbred populations, such as the Pima Indians of Arizona, USA, have a particularly high prevalence. This may be due to inherited factors, advantageous in times of famine, but in times of plenty result in obesity and hyperglycaemia.

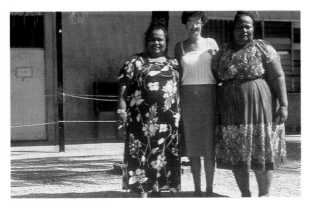

**Fig. 7** Two obese Nauruans with a health worker. These Pacific islanders have a very high prevalence of NIDDM.

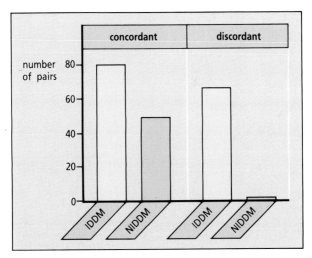

**Fig. 8** Twin data in IDDM and NIDDM. In identical twins with NIDDM, the concordance rate (i.e. with both twins in a pair having the condition) is almost 100%, implying the operation of strong genetic factors. In IDDM, the concordance rate is probably 33–50% implying not only the operation of genetic factors, but also of environmental agents. The figures shown here may provide an over-estimate of concordance as a result of a tendency to report concordant rather than discordant twin pairs. The discordance interval between members of a twin pair, that is the time between diagnosis of diabetes in the two subjects, is often remarkably short.

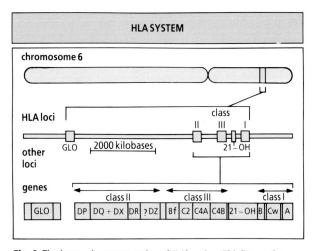

**Fig. 9** The human leucocyte antigen (HLA) region. This lies on the short arm of chromosome 6 and encodes the histocompatibility antigens and certain complement factors. HLA antigens are probably involved in self-recognition and the initiation of immune-mediated cell destruction. The prevalence of HLA-DR3 and DR4 is higher in diabetic than non-diabetic children and so these particular antigens convey increased risk for the development of diabetes. Polymorphism in the β chain of DQ may provide susceptibility to or protection from IDDM.

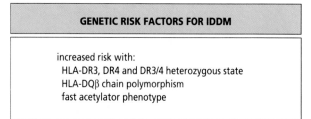

**Fig. 10** Genetic risk factors for IDDM. Apart from HLA, a variety of other genetic factors may be associated with IDDM. How they operate is currently unknown, but is under intense investigation.

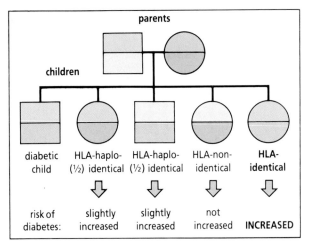

**Fig. 11** Multiplex family tree. When two or more children in the same family have diabetes, they are often of the same HLA type, which is inherited half from each parent. Thus, if a non-diabetic child has inherited the same HLA type as the diabetic child, it has a highly increased risk of developing the condition.

| ENVIRONMENTAL AGENTS POSSIBLY INVOLVED IN AETIOLOGY OF IDDM | |
|---|---|
| **viruses** | **toxins** |
| Coxsackie B4    rubella | chemicals? |
| mumps    reovirus | nitroso compounds? |

**Fig. 12** Aetiology of IDDM. Viruses have long been suspected as aetiological agents in IDDM due to a temporal association between viral infection and the appearance of hyperglycaemia. Although suspicion has fallen on Coxsackie, mumps and rubella, the vast majority of cases of diabetes do not seem to have a close antecedant viral infection. Pancreatic islets can be infected *in vitro* with viruses to cause cytolysis or chronic infection and laboratory animals can also be rendered diabetic by a range of viruses. Similarly, chemicals such as streptozotocin and alloxan can be used to produce diabetes in animals, but there is, as yet, little convincing evidence of chemical toxicity in human diabetes.

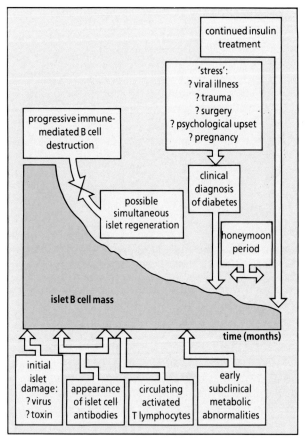

**Fig. 13** Pre-diabetic period in IDDM. In genetically predisposed individuals an environmental agent of unknown nature is presumed to cause the initial damage to the islets. This leads to a variety of immunological phenomena and an inflammatory reaction within the islets (insulitis). There is a gradual decline in insulin production which may be partly balanced by islet regeneration. At first, there is no metabolic disturbance, but when insulin production is reduced to approximately 10% of normal, coincidental stress may cause diabetes to appear. After a period of insulin treatment and the resolution of the incidental stress, islet function may recover and be sufficient to allow the temporary discontinuation of insulin injections, the 'honeymoon period'. With continued waning of insulin secretion, insulin injections become mandatory. Some authorities do not discontinue, but only reduce, insulin dosage in the honeymoon period.

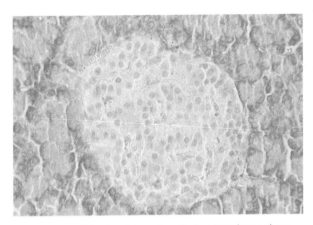

**Fig. 14** Normal islet. Insulin is produced in the islets of Langerhans. These endocrine glands are 75–175μm in diameter and number approximately $10^5$–$2 \times 10^6$ in the adult pancreas. Islet A cells secrete glucagon, B cells secrete insulin, D cells secrete somatostatin and PP cells secrete pancreatic polypeptide. The proportion of the different cells in each islet depends upon where the islet lies in the pancreas. In the islet-rich tail, insulin-secreting B cells form the core of the islets with a surrounding layer of A cells. H & E stain.

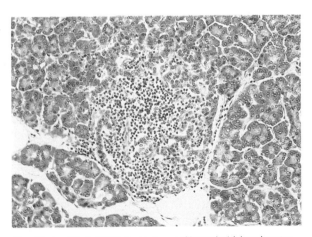

**Fig. 15** Insulitis. In IDDM, the islets are infiltrated with lymphocytes, mononuclear cells and polymorphs. This inflammatory reaction is termed 'insulitis'. It is unclear whether this is purely an autoimmune reaction or a response to islet damage by an unknown environmental agent. H & E stain.

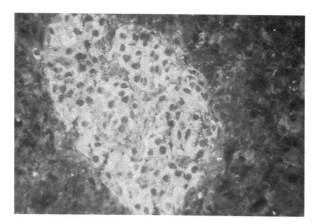

**Fig. 16** Islet cell antibodies. At the time of diagnosis, the sera of most IDDM subjects contain a variety of autoantibodies (islet cell antibodies; ICA) which react against islet cells. They have even been shown to be present before the clinical diagnosis of diabetes and, hence, may predict it. In most cases, for unknown reasons, ICA disappear within months of the clinical diagnosis of diabetes. Here 'classical' ICA are demonstrated by placing a drop of serum from a diabetic patient onto a section of pancreas from a blood group O donor and adding fluoresceinated anti-human IgG.

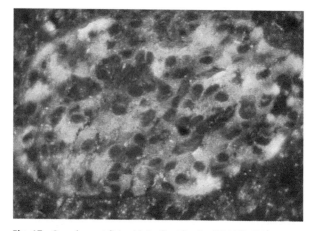

**Fig. 17** Complement-fixing islet cell antibodies (CF-ICA). CF-ICA are a powerful predictor of IDDM. They are demonstrated by adding the test serum, then fresh normal human serum as a source of complement and finally fluoresceinated anti-complement-C3.

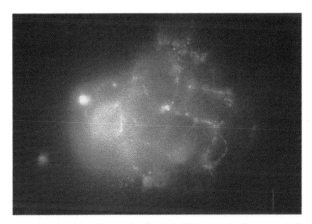

**Fig. 18** Islet cell surface antibodies (ICSA). ICSA may be demonstrated by immunofluorescent techniques, shown here with human fetal islets in monolayer culture. They may also predict the appearance of diabetes.

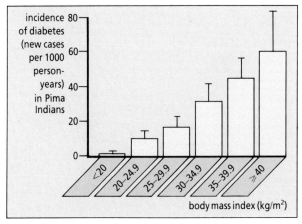

**Fig. 19** Association between obesity and diabetes. NIDDM is often associated with obesity, but it is important to realize that not all patients with NIDDM are obese and not all obese people are diabetic. Furthermore, IDDM may occur in the obese patient. Calorie restriction alone may be sufficient treatment to reduce the blood glucose level to normal in obese NIDDM patients. The mechanism by which obesity leads to diabetes is unknown; paradoxically, insulin levels may be higher than normal. Such hyperinsulinaemia must imply a defect in hormone action.

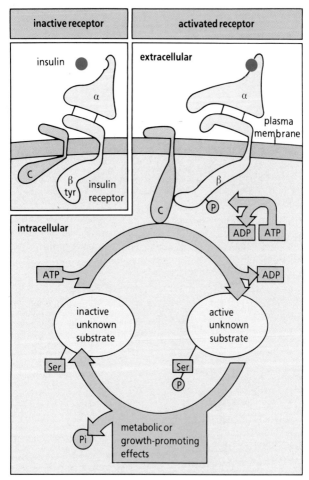

**Fig. 20** The insulin receptor. Insulin action may be compromised at the hormone receptor or there may be a subsequent post-receptor defect. The latter may be due to inefficiency or inadequate action of either internal cell messengers or signalling. In this theoretical diagram, the insulin receptor is represented as a tyrosine kinase. Association of insulin with its receptor causes a conformational change which allows the tyrosine kinase of the β-subunit to autophosphorylate one or more of its own tyrosine residues. The activated receptor as represented here, stimulates a separate kinase (C) in the membrane to phosphorylate a serine residue of an unknown cytoplasmic substrate. This change either activates or disinhibits insulin-sensitive intracellular pathways.

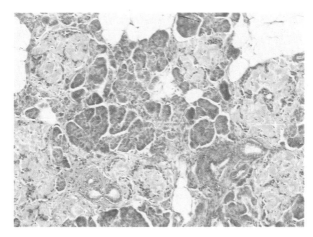

**Fig. 21**  Islet histology in NIDDM. This does not show any dramatic features. There is a general hyalinization of the islet, thought to represent senescence. Amyloid deposition, which is a feature of such islets, may have a pathogenic role. Gormori's chromium haematoxylin-phloxine stain.

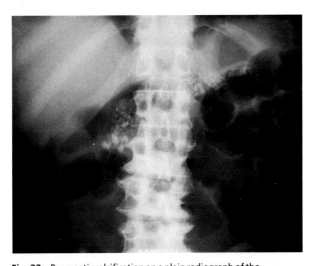

**Fig. 22**  Pancreatic calcification on a plain radiograph of the abdomen. This may suggest chronic pancreatic damage and is seen in some cases of diabetes in areas of Africa, the Indian sub-continent and the Far East. This patient from West Africa had IDDM and pancreatic exocrine insufficiency causing malabsorption.

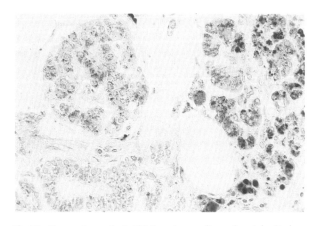

**Fig. 23**  Haemochromatosis. This iron storage disease is an inherited disorder and damages the pancreas, testes, heart, liver and pituitary. The associated staining of the skin led to the term 'bronzed diabetes'. Insulin treatment is usually required. Prussian blue staining reveals haemosiderin in islet endocrine cells (top left), duct epithelial cells (bottom left) and pancreatic acinar cells (right).

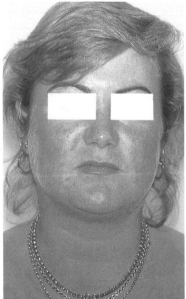

**Fig. 24**  Cushing's syndrome. This may be complicated by diabetes. Its features include a 'moon' face, 'buffalo hump', centripetal obesity, muscle wasting, striae, hypertension and psychological disturbances. It may be difficult to distinguish such a case from the many patients with simple obesity seen in the diabetic clinic. In addition to the usual symptoms and signs, diagnostic aids include 24h urinary cortisol excretion rate, and the overnight dexamethasone suppression test.

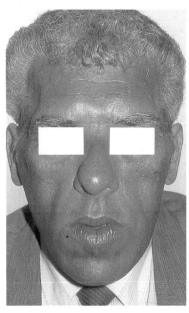

**Fig. 25** Acromegaly. Acromegalic patients may develop diabetes as growth hormone is an antagonist of insulin. Its treatment depends upon the degree of metabolic disturbance. In acromegaly, the GTT is performed with simultaneous measurement of growth hormone levels; they are not suppressed by hyperglyceamia.

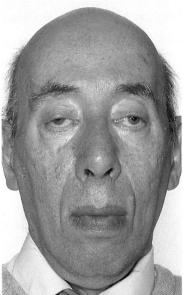

**Fig. 26** Dystrophia myotonica in a 61-year-old man. The disorder was diagnosed at age 40 years and he was found to have diabetes at age 54 years. His myopathic appearance and ptosis are typical of this condition.

# TREATMENT: DIET

The treatment of diabetes can be divided into three categories: diet alone, diet with oral hypoglycaemic agents and diet plus insulin. Thus, diet is the cornerstone of all treatments for diabetes; its importance cannot be stressed enough. Prescription of the diet starts with a detailed assessment of the patient's usual eating habits, taking account of lifestyle, work patterns and culture. Each patient requires an individually tailored diet plan according to his or her needs. Currently fashionable advice includes: not restricting carbohydrate intake, but altering the type consumed; increasing dietary fibre; and reducing saturated fat intake.

The assessment of obesity or the reverse is important and is simple using the formula for body mass index (BMI): (weight in kilograms)/(height in metres)$^2$. BMI is graded as follows: 20–24.9, normal; 25–29.9, grade I obesity; 30–40, grade II obesity; 40+, grade III obesity.

| PRINCIPLES OF DIETARY TREATMENT |
| --- |
| **NIDDM** |
| 1. Obese patients: reduce weight<br>2. Non-obese patients: follow diet low in refined carbohydrate (possibly increase unrefined carbohydrate) |
| **IDDM** |
| 1. Total daily calorie intake takes into account:<br>   (i) desired body weight<br>   (ii) energy expenditure (assessment of daily activities)<br>   (iii) growth (children)<br>   (iv) extra requirement, e.g. pregnancy and breast feeding<br>2. Distribution of carbohydrate intake:<br>   (i) system of food exchanges based on 10g portions<br>   (ii) individual diet plan based on personal daily routine |
| **All patients** |
| 1. Avoid easily absorbed refined carbohydrates; take unrefined<br>2. Emphasize dietary fibre<br>3. Reduce saturated fat; substitute polyunsaturated fat<br>4. Take alcohol in moderation |

**Fig. 27** Principles of dietary treatment.

## DIET PLAN BASED ON 10g CARBOHYDRATE FOOD EXCHANGES

| Meals | Carbohydrate | | Examples |
|---|---|---|---|
| | Exchanges | Grams | |
| breakfast | 5 | 50 | branflakes, toast, tea |
| snack | 1 | 10 | banana, coffee |
| lunch | 4 | 40 | cheese salad, sandwich, fruit, tea |
| snack | 1 | 10 | biscuits, tea |
| dinner | 5 | 50 | avocado or vegetable soup, steak, potatoes, vegetables, fruit |
| snack | 1.5 | 15 | wholemeal toast, coffee |
| daily milk | 1.5 | 15 | 300ml |
| total | 19 | 190 | |

**Fig. 28** Diet plan for use primarily in insulin-dependent patients utilizing the concept of 'food exchanges' based on portions, each containing 10g carbohydrate. This allows variation in meal menus, while keeping the daily carbohydrate total and its distribution relatively constant.

| CHOICE OF CARBOHYDRATE | |
|---|---|
| **Encourage** | **Discourage** |

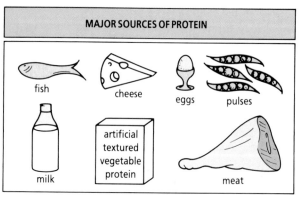

**Fig. 29** Carbohydrates. Up to 60% of the daily diet may be taken as carbohydrate. Refined foods contain sugars which are easily absorbed and may worsen glycaemic control if taken in excess. Complexed unrefined carbohydrates are less readily absorbed and may make less impact upon blood glucose levels. They also tend to contain natural fibre, an increase in which is desirable.

**MAJOR SOURCES OF PROTEIN**

**Fig. 30** Proteins. In developed countries, the daily protein intake is about 60–120g, although less may be sufficient and may retard the progression of renal damage in patients with early nephropathy. To reduce saturated fat consumption, chicken and leaner cuts of meat are preferable, as are sources of vegetable protein, such as pulses and textured soya protein, which may also increase dietary fibre.

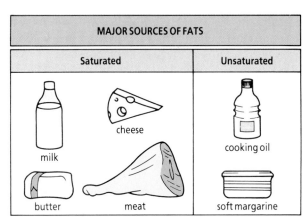

| MAJOR SOURCES OF FATS | |
|---|---|
| Saturated | Unsaturated |
| milk  cheese  butter  meat | cooking oil  soft margarine |

**Fig. 31**  Fats. With previous dietary advice, fat consumption often increased to compensate for the reduced intake of carbohydrate. Because atheromatous vascular disease is an important long-term complication of diabetes and patients with poorly controlled diabetes may have raised plasma lipid levels, current opinion favours a general reduction in fat intake. Saturated fats should be decreased and replaced with unsaturated ones. Simple measures include changing from butter to a low fat spread, avoiding cream and dairy products with a high fat content and having skimmed milk.

| ENERGY CONTENT OF ALCOHOLIC DRINKS | | | |
|---|---|---|---|
| | Carbohydrate (kcal) | Alcohol (kcal) | Total (kcal) |
| ½ pint beer | 28 | 56 | 84 |
| 1 glass wine | 20 | 56 | 76 |
| 1 measure spirits | 0 | 56 | 56 |

**Fig. 32**  Alcohol. This is not prohibited in the diabetic diet, although it is best taken in moderation. Patients should be made aware that it is a rich source of calories at 7kcals/g, may potentiate hypoglycaemia and may cause facial flushing in patients taking sulphonylureas.

## TREATMENT: ORAL HYPOGLYCAEMIC AGENTS

Diet treatment alone for NIDDM may fail for two broad reasons: inadequate adherence to the dietary advice or because the metabolic derangement is too severe to be corrected by diet alone. Once it has been decided that diet alone has failed, oral hypoglycaemic agents should be considered. Before beginning treatment with them, it is important to explain to the patient that: (i) they are not a substitute for dietary treatment; and (ii) the dietary treatment must be continued along with the tablets. Patients often wrongly believe that their diet may be relaxed or abandoned with the introduction of tablets. It is a disservice to tell patients they have 'mild diabetes' because they are taking tablets and not insulin injections. Such a misnomer may produce a false sense of security, leading to complacent inattention to diabetes. Non-insulin-dependent diabetes in time may lead to the whole spectrum of chronic complications.

Three types of oral hypoglycaemic agents are available: sulphonylureas, biguanides and alpha-glucosidase inhibitors, although the latter are strictly antihyperglycaemic rather than hypoglycaemic in effect. Guar gum preparations help slow carbohydrate digestion and absorption.

| ORAL HYPOGLYCAEMIC AGENTS | | |
| --- | --- | --- |
| | **Sulphonylureas** | **Biguanides** |
| **Mechanisms of action** | enhance endogenous insulin secretion<br><br>probable extra-pancreatic effects | decrease appetite<br><br>reduce intestinal glucose absorption<br><br>decrease gluconeogenesis<br><br>increase anaerobic glycolysis<br><br>increase muscle glucose uptake |
| **Indications** | diet has failed in non-obese NIDDM patient | diet has failed in NIDDM patient, particularly if obese |

**Fig. 33** Features of oral hypoglycaemic agents. If the maximal dose of one type is reached, then the other may be added if desired.

| SULPHONYLUREAS | | | | |
|---|---|---|---|---|
| **Name** | **Duration of action (hours)** | **Dosage range (mg)** | **Tablet size (mg)** | **Special features** |
| **first generation** | | | | |
| tolbutamide | 6–8 | 500–3000 | 250, 500 | |
| chlorpropamide | 36+ | 100–500 | 100, 250 | avoid in elderly or in renal failure |
| tolazamide | 12–24 | 100–750 | 100,250 | |
| acetohexamide | 12–18 | 500–1500 | 250,500 | |
| **second generation** | | | | |
| glibenclamide | 5–20 | 2.5–20 | 2.5, 5 | |
| glipizide | 5–12 | 2.5–45 | 2.5, 5 | |
| glibornuride | 5–12 | 12.5–75 | 12.5 | |
| gliclazide | 5–20 | 40–320 | 80 | antiplatelet action |
| gliquidone | 5 | 15–180 | 30 | useful in renal failure |
| **related compound** glymidine | 12–24 | 500–2000 | 500 | no cross–allergenicity |

**Fig. 34** Characteristics of the sulphonylureas. All are metabolized in the liver, but only slightly in the case of chlorpropamide.

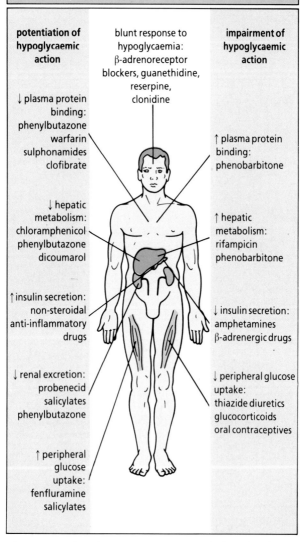

## DRUG INTERACTIONS WITH SULPHONYLUREAS

**potentiation of hypoglycaemic action**

blunt response to hypoglycaemia: β-adrenoreceptor blockers, guanethidine, reserpine, clonidine

**impairment of hypoglycaemic action**

↓ plasma protein binding:
phenylbutazone
warfarin
sulphonamides
clofibrate

↑ plasma protein binding:
phenobarbitone

↓ hepatic metabolism:
chloramphenicol
phenylbutazone
dicoumarol

↑ hepatic metabolism:
rifampicin
phenobarbitone

↑ insulin secretion:
non-steroidal anti-inflammatory drugs

↓ insulin secretion:
amphetamines
β-adrenergic drugs

↓ renal excretion:
probenecid
salicylates
phenylbutazone

↓ peripheral glucose uptake:
thiazide diuretics
glucocorticoids
oral contraceptives

↑ peripheral glucose uptake:
fenfluramine
salicylates

**Fig. 35** Apart from drug interactions, unwanted effects of sulphonylureas include hypoglycaemia, facial flushing with alcohol, skin rashes, anorexia, nausea, jaundice, exfoliative dermatitis and blood dyscrasias. Apart from hypoglycaemia, they are all uncommon.

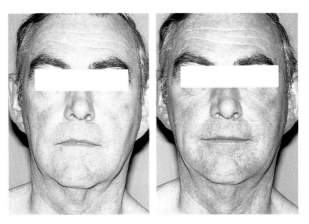

**Fig. 36** Alcohol flush. Facial appearance of a patient on chlorpropamide before and after taking alcohol. A pronounced facial flush can be seen.

| METFORMIN | |
|---|---|
| tablet sizes: | 500mg, 850mg |
| dosage: | up to 3g daily in divided doses usually before meals |
| metabolism: | protein-bound; renal excretion |
| contra-indications: | renal, cardiac and hepatic impairment; other diabetic complications (relative) |
| unwanted effects: | lactic acidosis (rare), abdominal discomfort, flatulence, diarrhoea, folate and vitamin $B_{12}$ malabsorption |

**Fig. 37a** Metformin is the main biguanide used at present; phenformin has been associated with lactic acidosis, although this is rare, and has been withdrawn.

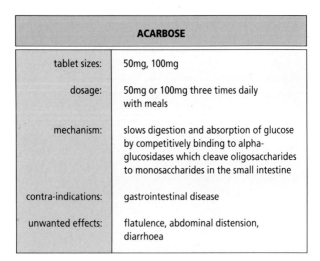

| ACARBOSE | |
|---|---|
| tablet sizes: | 50mg, 100mg |
| dosage: | 50mg or 100mg three times daily with meals |
| mechanism: | slows digestion and absorption of glucose by competitively binding to alpha-glucosidases which cleave oligosaccharides to monosaccharides in the small intestine |
| contra-indications: | gastrointestinal disease |
| unwanted effects: | flatulence, abdominal distension, diarrhoea |

**Fig. 37b** Acarbose is a non-absorbed inhibitor of carbohydrate digestion.

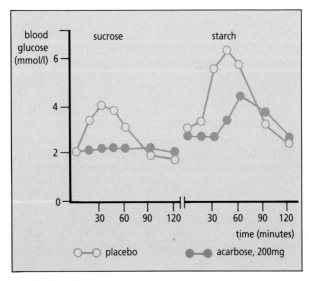

**Fig. 37c** Peaks in blood glucose levels after a meal are lowered by the addition of acarbose 200mg compared with placebo. Acarbose blocks alpha-glucosidase enzymes and so inhibits carbohydrate digestion. Adapted from Jenkins 1981.

# TREATMENT: INSULIN

Since its discovery in 1922, insulin has provided life-saving treatment for millions of diabetic people around the world. Physicians who are not specialists in diabetes often find the management of insulin therapy perplexing because of the lack of a finite dosage scale and the bewildering variety of insulins available. Familiarity with a few different insulins and regimens is more helpful for the non-specialist than trying to be an expert on all aspects of insulin treatment.

The aims of insulin treatment are:
- To control blood glucose and disordered metabolism.
- To avoid hyperglycaemia and hypoglycaemia.
- To achieve satisfactory growth in children.
- To achieve and maintain normal body weight.

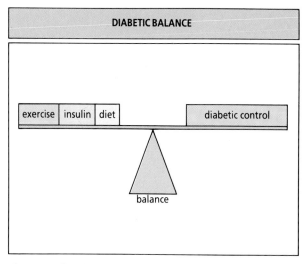

**Fig. 38** Diabetic balance. The control of diabetes depends upon the interplay between diet, insulin and exercise.

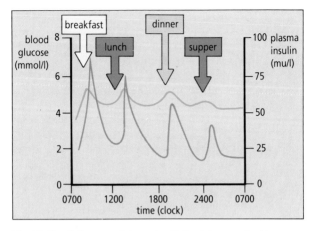

**Fig. 39** Blood glucose and plasma insulin levels in normal subjects. Blood glucose is kept strictly within the normal range (approximately 2.5–7.5mmol/l) no matter what or how much is consumed. Insulin is secreted not only in response to meals (prandial boosts), but also between meals (basal insulin secretion). When planning insulin treatment, it is important to mimic not only the prandial boosts, but also to provide a constant background availability of insulin representing basal secretion.

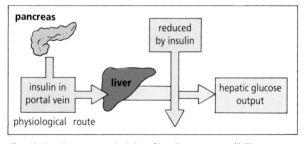

**Fig. 40** Two important principles of insulin treatment. (i) The physiological route of insulin secretion from the pancreas is via the portal vein to the liver. In the liver, approximately 50% of the insulin secreted is used to control hepatic metabolism, including hepatic glucose output. Therapeutic insulin given subcutaneously is delivered by a non-physiological route; it first enters the peripheral circulation, only later reaching the liver. (ii) Without insulin, hepatic glucose output rises, which explains why fasting blood glucose levels may be elevated in an insulin-deficient patient. Therefore, the liver must be constantly under the influence of insulin and this should be considered when designing an insulin regimen.

## Understanding the wide range of insulins

There are many different insulins available and they tend to
be prescribed by brand name, unlike most other drugs.
Many insulins are identical to each other or very similar. To
help understanding, any insulin can be classified according
to its length of action, which defines how frequently it
should be given, and its species of origin.

| TYPES OF INSULIN | | | |
|---|---|---|---|
| Approx. length of action (hours) | Frequency of injections/day | Type | Examples |
| short:   4–6 | 2–4 | soluble | Actrapid Velosulin Humulin S |
| medium:   12 | 2 | isophane | Insulatard Protaphane Humulin I |
|  |  | insulin zinc suspension | Monotard |
| long:   24–30 | 1 | insulin zinc suspension | Human Ultratard |

**Fig. 41** Classification of insulins. All insulins may be broadly classified
as either short-, medium- or long-acting. This provides information on
how frequently they should be injected.

| Animal insulin | Difference to human insulin |
|----------------|------------------------------|
| cow | 3 amino acids |
| pig | 1 amino acid |

| Human insulin | Method of manufacture |
|---------------|------------------------|
| biosynthetic | DNA coding for human insulin instructs manufacture in *Escherichia coli* bacteria |
| semisynthetic | porcine insulin is enzymatically modified to make it identical to human insulin |

**Fig. 42** Sources of insulin. Insulin was originally obtained from the pancreas of pigs and cattle from slaughterhouses. Today there is an increasing trend towards the use of human insulin. This is currently made by two routes: biosynthetic, in DNA-directed *E. coli* and semisynthetic by enzymatically modifying porcine insulin. Human identical insulins are less antigenic than animal insulins, but have no other proven important advantages.

| Insulin | | Morning dose | Evening dose |
|---------|--------|--------------|--------------|
| | Proportion | 2/3 | 1/3 |
| Taken as: | short | 1/3 | 1/3 |
| | medium | 2/3 | 2/3 |
| example: | short | 8 | 4 |
| | medium | 16 | 8 |
| | **total** = 36 units | 24 | 12 |

**Fig. 43** General dosage regimen. Many patients can be stabilized with a regimen of twice-daily injections, each consisting of a mixture of short- and medium-acting insulins, given in the proportions shown here. To optimize control from the starting doses, each of the four doses can be adjusted, making it a flexible regimen. If the evening injection does not last until the next morning, it may be split, giving the short-acting component before the evening meal and the medium-acting at bedtime. Fixed-ratio mixtures provide a further simplification of the twice-daily regimen. They contain a short- and a medium-acting insulin ready mixed and are available in ratios from 10% to 50% soluble with correspondingly 90% to 50% isophane.

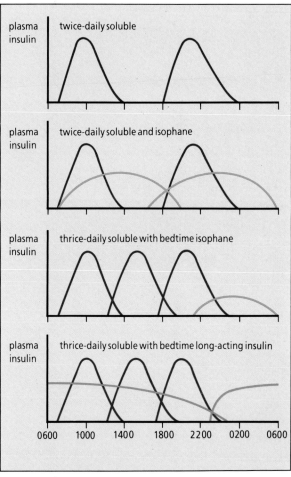

**Fig. 44** Designing an insulin regimen; the effect on plasma insulin concentrations of various regimens, shown diagrammatically and idealized. The regimen should be selected to suit the lifestyle and requirements of the individual patient, bearing in mind age, weight, work and daily routine. The dose of insulin is empirical; it is that required to optimize blood glucose levels throughout the 24h period. An average dose would be 30–40 (range 2 to several 100) units/day or 0.75units/kg body weight. Hypoglycaemia suggests a reduction and hyperglycaemia suggests an increase in the dose of the insulin acting at that time. Residual endogenous insulin secretion may enable a lower insulin dose.

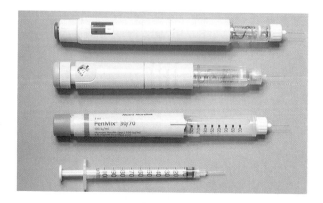

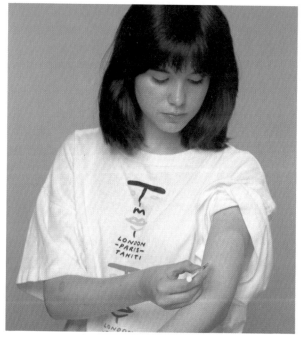

**Fig. 45** Plastic disposable syringes have simplified injection equipment. Use of multiple daily pre-prandial soluble insulin injections given by cartridge pen (e.g. Novopen, upper; Becton Dickinson pen, second down) with a bedtime medium- or long-acting insulin is becoming more common. Preloaded disposable insulin pens are available (third down). With modern equipment, injections (lower) are simple and almost painless.

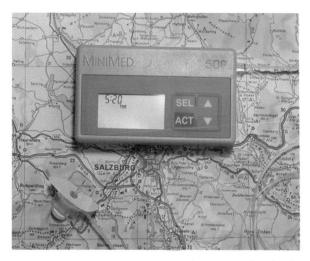

**Fig. 46** Insulin infusion pump. This is a device which provides a basal supply of insulin and pre-prandial boosts, a regimen called continuous subcutaneous insulin infusion (CSII). The Minimed infusion pump illustrated here is small and may be worn on a belt or in a pocket. It drives a syringe within it to provide continuous delivery of subcutaneous insulin at basal rates with pre-meal boosts. This type of treatment can provide very tight control of blood glucose levels.

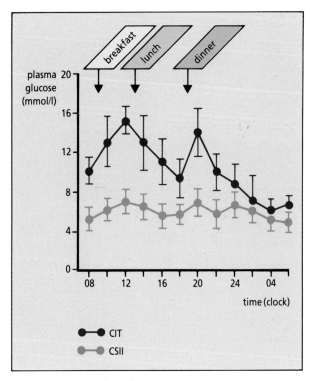

**Fig. 47** Comparison of circadian plasma glucose levels during treatment with conventional insulin treatment (CIT) and continuous subcutaneous insulin infusion (CSII). Circadian plasma glucose concentrations were measured in nine insulin-dependent diabetic patients who were treated in random order by either CIT or CSII. The period of CSII therapy was three weeks. Values represent mean and SEM calculated from a day profile performed in hospital on each regimen.

# GLYCAEMIC CONTROL AND ITS ASSESSMENT

## The importance of glycaemic control

Before the introduction of insulin, diabetes often proved fatal. After its introduction, although patients were kept alive for much longer, they still had a shortened life span and it was found that they developed a variety of chronic complications. During the first fifty years of effective treatment, it was unclear whether a straightforward relationship existed between chronic hyperglycaemia and the development of complications and, therefore, whether tight control of the blood glucose level would prevent the development of complications. Clinical experience showed that some patients with apparently good control developed complications, while others with poor control did not. Resolution of this issue was hampered by several factors: before the use of glycosylated proteins as an index of glycaemia, there was difficulty in assessing control; most studies were retrospective and not prospective; and groups of patients with varying degrees of poor control were compared.

Current opinion holds that there is a relationship between chronic hyperglycaemia and the development of long-term complications. Research on this aspect has been aided by the ability to virtually normalize blood glucose levels by pump treatment (see page 45) and prospectively compare the effect of this on the development or progression of complications with that of conventional treatments producing less tight control. The diabetes control and complications trial (DCCT) in the USA clearly showed that tight glycaemic control provided by intensive insulin treatment in IDDM patients over 9 years dramatically reduced the appearance and progression of diabetic complications. Each diabetic patient has to assume day-to-day supervision and adjustment of his or her condition and becomes, to some extent, physician, nurse, dietitian and laboratory technician.

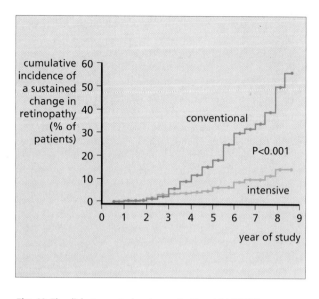

**Fig. 48** The diabetes control and complications trial (DCCT) prospectively examined the relationship between glycaemic control and the development and progression of long-term complications. 1441 insulin-dependent diabetic patients (726 with no retinopathy and 715 with mild retinopathy) were randomised to either intensive therapy with three or more injections per day or pumped insulin thereby aiming for tight control, or conventional therapy with one or two injections per day. Intensive therapy reduced the mean risk of the onset of retinopathy by 76% during the course of the nine-year study.

| ASSESSMENT OF GLYCAEMIC CONTROL | |
|---|---|
| **Home** | **Hospital** |
| urinalysis<br>blood glucose estimation | glycosylated protein:<br>  haemoglobin<br>  albumin<br>  hair<br>fructosamine |

**Fig. 49**  Methods of assessment of glycaemic control.

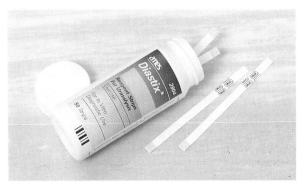

**Fig. 50** Urine test strips. These are simple, cheap and convenient. The appearance of glucose in the urine depends on the blood glucose level exceeding the individual's renal glucose threshold. The semi-quantitative result may be influenced by the timing of the specimen tested and the last voiding of urine. Urine testing provides too little information to adjust an insulin regimen accurately.

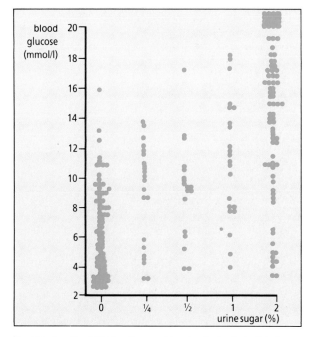

**Fig. 51** Results of 250 simultaneous blood and urine tests. This shows how inaccurately urine tests reflect blood glucose levels.

## Home blood glucose monitoring

The introduction of reagent strips for the measurement of blood glucose at home has enabled patients to document their level of glycaemic control more accurately and has provided better information for the self-adjustment of the treatment regimen. A drop of blood is drawn from a finger tip (the side is less painful than the front) or ear-lobe, preferably using a spring-loaded device. The blood is dropped on to a reagent pad containing a glucose-oxidase system which changes colour according to the blood glucose level. The colour change may be read quantitatively in a reflectance meter which gives a read-out of the blood glucose level.

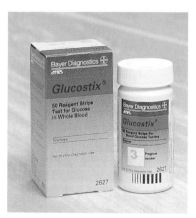

**Fig. 52** Example of reagent strips used to measure blood glucose.

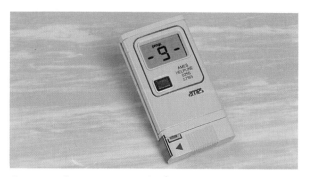

**Fig. 53** A reflectance meter may be used to read the colour change on blood glucose reagent strips. The more advanced ones incorporate a memory and the ability to generate a printout and statistical analysis.

## Assessment of medium-term glycaemic control

Glucose becomes non-enzymatically attached to many body proteins; the higher the blood glucose level, the more is attached. By measuring the percentage of total protein, for example haemoglobin, which has glucose attached (glycosylated or glycated), an indication of mean glycaemic control over the preceding two to three months is provided. Glycosylated haemoglobin ($HbA_1$ or $HbA_{1c}$) can be detected by a variety of methods including column chromatography, isoelectric focusing and colorimetry.

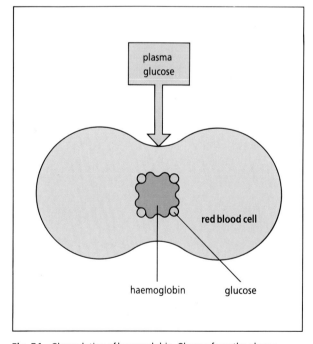

**Fig. 54** Glycosylation of haemoglobin. Glucose from the plasma enters red blood cells and attaches non-enzymatically to haemoglobin. In non-diabetic subjects, about 4–8% of haemoglobin is glycosylated (the precise normal range depending upon method), whereas it is increasingly higher in diabetic subjects with poor glycaemic control. Measurement of serum fructosamine is rapid, simple, reproducible and provides a shorter term assessment of glycaemic control than $HbA_{1c}$.

# DIABETIC COMPLICATIONS: AN OVERVIEW

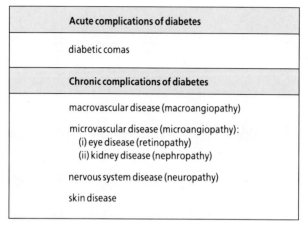

| Acute complications of diabetes |
| --- |
| diabetic comas |
| **Chronic complications of diabetes** |
| macrovascular disease (macroangiopathy) |
| microvascular disease (microangiopathy): <br> (i) eye disease (retinopathy) <br> (ii) kidney disease (nephropathy) |
| nervous system disease (neuropathy) |
| skin disease |

**Fig. 55** Diabetic complications. Diabetic patients may develop a wide variety of complications. The physician caring for them requires a broad knowledge of medicine, encompassing clinical biochemistry, vascular disease, ophthalmology, nephrology, neurology, dermatology and psychology. Although long-term complications usually take years to develop, they may be present at the diagnosis of NIDDM, as chronic hyperglycaemia may have been present prior to diagnosis.

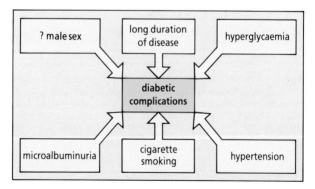

**Fig. 56** Risk factors for the development and progression of diabetic complications. The most powerful risk factor is hyperglycaemia, the effect of which depends upon its degree and duration. Hypertension, if untreated, hastens the progression of nephropathy, while cigarette smoking is a risk factor for macroangiopathy. Male sex may predispose to microangiopathy. The role of genetic factors remains speculative.

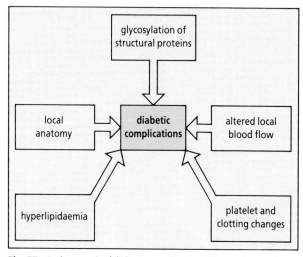

**Fig. 57** Pathogenesis of diabetic complications. The precise way in which the diabetic state produces its chronic complications is unknown. There may be one or several different mechanisms involved. The anatomical site of the lesion has some importance, for example the structure of the retina may allow the growth of new vessels, while hydrostatic forces may favour atheromatous change in the lower as opposed to upper limbs. Glycosylation of structural proteins may lead to physico-chemical changes, such as opacification of the lens causing cataract, thickening of the glomerular basement membrane seen in nephropathy, and alterations in collagen leading to limited joint mobility (cheiroarthropathy) and Dupuytren's contracture. Micro- and macroangiopathy may result from a combination of these and local alterations in blood flow (both increased and decreased), an increase in plasma viscosity and changes in platelets, clotting factors and lipids.

# DIABETIC COMPLICATIONS: COMAS

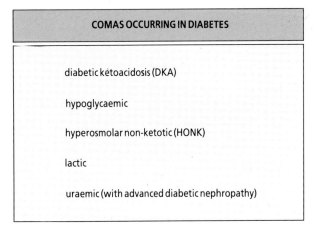

**Fig. 58** Four main types of comas occur in diabetes. They all require immediate treatment.

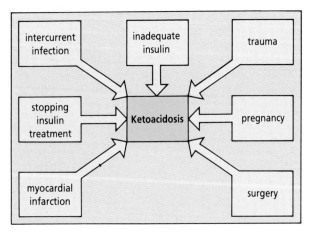

**Fig. 59** Ketoacidosis. Patients with IDDM require daily insulin injections; if missed or stopped, ketoacidosis may develop. In the presence of intercurrent illness or metabolic 'stress', insulin requirements are increased and thus the dose should be raised. If it is not raised, there is relative insulin deficiency, which may also predispose to ketoacidosis.

**PRESENTATION OF DIABETIC KETOACIDOSIS**

| Symptoms | Signs |
|----------|-------|
| vomiting (70%) | tachycardia |
| thirst (55%) | hypotension |
| polyuria (40%) | dehydration |
| weight loss (20%) | warm, dry skin |
| abdominal pain (15%) | hyperventilation |
| weakness (20%) | hypothermia |
|  | impaired consciousness |

**Fig. 60** Symptoms and signs of diabetic ketoacidosis. These develop over hours or days and reflect dehydration, hyperglycaemia, metabolic acidosis and the precipitating cause. The frequency with which symptoms occur is shown.

**INVESTIGATION IN DIABETIC KETOACIDOSIS**

| Assessment of severity | Establishing cause |
|------------------------|--------------------|
| glucose | careful physical examination |
| urea and electrolytes | chest radiograph |
| full blood count, packed cell volume and white cell count | ECG |
| blood gases, including pH and bicarbonate | blood and urine cultures |
| blood ketones | throat swab |

**Fig. 61** Initial investigations in diabetic ketoacidosis. These provide a baseline assessment of the severity of the condition and aim to establish its cause.

| FLUID REPLACEMENT REGIMEN |
|---|
| use normal saline (0.9% NaCl; 150mmol/l)<br><br>1st hour: 1.5 litres<br>2nd hour: 1.0 litre<br>3rd & 4th hours: 1.0 litre over 2 hours<br>5th hour onwards: 2.0 litres every 8 hours<br><br>change to 5% or 10% dextrose, 1.0 litre 8 hourly when rehydrated<br>and blood glucose falls to 12mmol/l<br><br>monitor state of hydration throughout |

**Fig. 62** Treatment of ketoacidosis. Patients with diabetic ketoacidosis are severely dehydrated and require large volumes of replacement fluid intravenously. Normal saline is used initially and is then replaced with 5% or 10% dextrose when the blood glucose level falls to approximately 12mmol/l. Elderly patients may develop fluid overload if treated too vigorously. Central venous pressure monitoring is helpful.

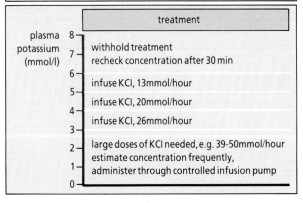

**Fig. 63** Recommended regimen for potassium replacement in ketoacidosis. Plasma potassium may be high initially but fall to normal and then below normal during treatment. Frequent potassium measurements are required and replacement is started when the level falls to within the normal range.

| INSULIN REPLACEMENT |
| --- |
| **Continuous intravenous infusion (soluble insulin)** |
| children: 0.1u/kg/h<br>adults: 6u/h |
| **Intermittent intramuscular infusion** |
| children: 0.25u/kg at once, then 0.1u/kg/h<br>adults: 20u at once, then 6 – 10u/h |

**Fig. 64** Insulin replacement regimens. Continuous low-dose intravenous insulin by an infusion pump readily reduces severe hyperglycaemia. When the blood glucose level reaches approximately 12mmol/l, the pump rate may be reduced to 1–2u/h in adults. Constant supervision is required to prevent technical problems, such as pump disconnection from the intravenous lines. The pump should never be switched off, as the patient will quickly reverse into ketoacidosis. If the blood glucose level falls too low, intravenous or oral glucose should be given. As a useful alternative to pumped intravenous insulin, intermittent (e.g. hourly) intramuscular insulin can be given.

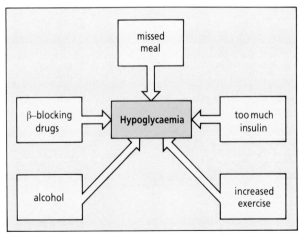

**Fig. 65** Precipitants of hypoglycaemia. Hypoglycaemia may occur in patients taking sulphonylureas as well as those on insulin treatment.

| HYPOGLYCAEMIA SIGNS | |
|---|---|
| **Symptoms** | **Signs** |
| subjective sensation e.g. 'light headed' | altered conscious level (appears intoxicated, abnormal behaviour and coma) |
| sweating | |
| palpitations | tachycardia |
| circumoral tingling | diplopia |
| hunger | pallor |
| blurred vision | tremor |
| | motor disturbance |

**Fig. 66** Symptoms and signs of hypoglycaemia.

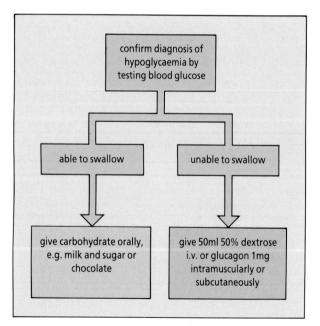

**Fig. 67** Management of hypoglycaemia. A clinical diagnosis is sufficient if the blood glucose level cannot be confirmed rapidly. The subsequent management depends upon the consciousness level and the ability to swallow.

## HONK: RISK FACTORS

old age

NIDDM

taking glucose-containing drinks, e.g. cola and lemonade

antihypertensive medication

surgery

infection

**Fig. 68** Risk factors for hyperosmolar non-ketotic coma (HONK). Why ketosis does not develop is unclear, although patients with HONK may have sufficient insulin secretion to prevent the development of ketosis but not to prevent the development of severe hyperglycaemia.

## HONK: FEATURES

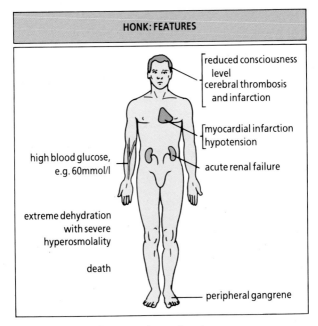

reduced consciousness level
cerebral thrombosis and infarction

myocardial infarction
hypotension

high blood glucose, e.g. 60mmol/l

acute renal failure

extreme dehydration with severe hyperosmolality

death

peripheral gangrene

**Fig. 69** Features of hyperosmolar non-ketotic coma.

**HONK: MANAGEMENT**

fluid replacement: i.v. normal (0.9%) or half normal (0.45%) saline

insulin: low-dose i.v. infusion or intermittent i.m. injections

potassium replacements: according to plasma K$^+$

anticoagulants: heparin and/or prostacyclin infusions

**Fig. 70**  Management of hyperosmolar non-ketotic coma.

**LACTIC ACIDOSIS**

**occurrence:** rare; usually older patients

**precipitants:** biguanides (especially phenformin)
metabolic acidosis: renal, cardiac or liver failure
septic shock

**features:** metabolic acidosis with high plasma lactate
(normal 0.4–1.0 mmol/l)
hypotension
dehydration

**management:** treatment of underlying cause
i.v. NaHCO$_3$

**outcome:** often fatal

**Fig. 71**  Aspects of lactic acidosis.

## LONG-TERM COMPLICATIONS: MACROANGIOPATHY

Atheromatous disease is common in diabetes, although it probably has the same aetiopathogenesis as in non-diabetic subjects. Patients with poorly controlled diabetes have hyperlipidaemia which may be a predisposing factor. Older-style diets often suggested a replacement of carbohydrate by fat, for example cheese or milk, which may lead to increased lipid levels. Hypertension which contributes to vascular disease is common in long-duration diabetes and may help explain the complex inerrelationship between diabetes, renal impairment and atheromatous disease. In addition to local stenosis of medium-sized arteries, which may be alleviated by surgery or angioplasty, there may also be microvascular changes which are less amenable to treatment. Diabetic patients should be advised not to smoke because it may further contribute to their risk of vascular disease. Treatment of diabetes, hyperlipidaemia and hypertension may reduce cardiovascular risk.

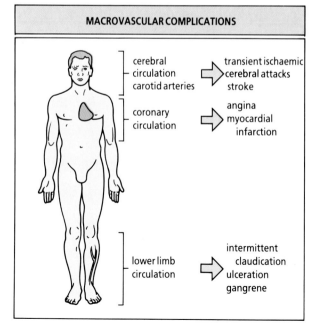

**Fig. 72** Macrovascular complications.

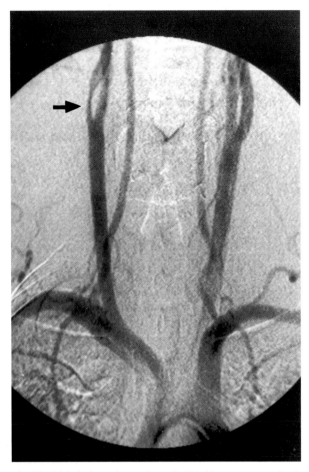

**Fig. 73** Digital subtraction angiography (DSA) is a computer-assisted technique used to enhance vascular imaging. Atheromatous disease of the carotid or cerebral arteries may lead to transient ischaemic attacks, amaurosis fugax and completed strokes. If angiography shows a lesion amenable to surgery, endarterectomy may prevent permanent neurological deficit. Medical management includes aspirin and dipyridamole. This diabetic man developed a right central retinal artery occlusion and intermittent attacks of paraesthesiae affecting the left side of his body. The DSA shows a profound narrowing of the right internal carotid artery just distal to the bifurcation (arrowed) which was alleviated by carotid endarterectomy.

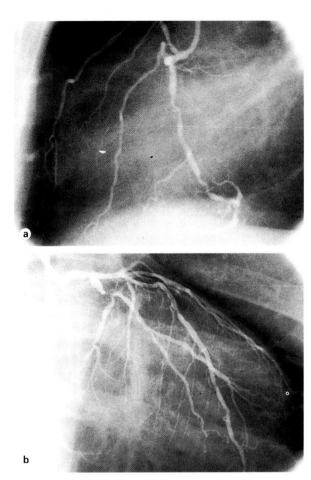

**Fig. 74** Coronary angiogram. Angina and myocardial infarction are common in patients with diabetes. In addition to segmental coronary artery stenosis, there may be diffuse small vessel disease which is not readily amenable to by-pass surgery or angioplasty. These frames are from the cine angiogram of a diabetic man with severe angina and show proximal stenoses and multiple diffuse irregularities. (a) The right coronary angiogram (right lateral projection) shows multiple critical stenoses with generalized and diffuse mural irregularity. (b) The left coronary angiogram (right anterior oblique projection) shows severe proximal stenosis and diffuse distal disease involving both the anterior descending and circumflex arteries.

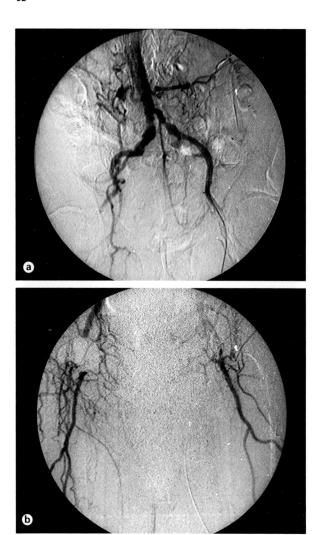

**Fig. 75**  Peripheral vascular disease. Intermittent claudication, ulceration and gangrene may be manifestations of peripheral vascular disease. Angiography may reveal a localized block amenable to surgery. DSA films of an elderly man with a necrotic toe reveal (a) bilateral common iliac stenoses and (b) almost complete occlusion of the common femoral arteries bilaterally at the level of the hip joints, with filling of the profunda arteries by collateral vessels and no filling of the superficial femoral arteries.

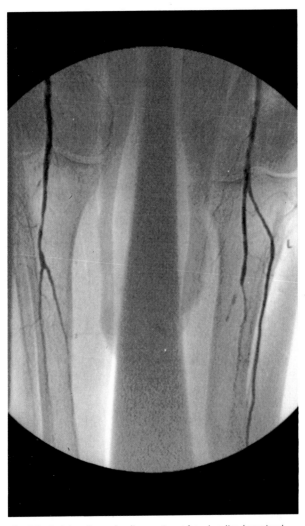

**Fig. 76** Peripheral vascular disease. Apart from localized proximal stenoses, generally poor distal circulation is a common problem in diabetic patients. Unlike the former, poor distal circulation is more difficult to treat and may eventually necessitate local amputation. This DSA shows poor peripheral circulation past the popliteal arteries bilaterally.

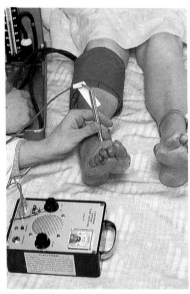

**Fig. 77** Doppler machine. Palpation of the peripheral pulses is often difficult. Doppler ultrasound location and pressure measurements give helpful information. Reduced blood flow is indicated by a dorsalis pedis systolic/brachial systolic pressure ratio of < 0.9. A ratio of 0.5 indicates poor blood flow and 0.25 usually indicates the need for surgery.

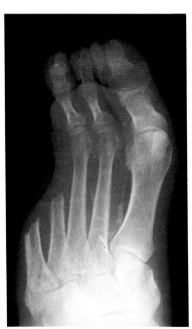

**Fig. 78** Digital calcification. Calcification of the digital arteries of the foot is a sign of underlying vascular disease and is seen particularly in patients with renal impairment. This patient has had amputations of the fourth and fifth toes through the metatarsals because of gangrene.

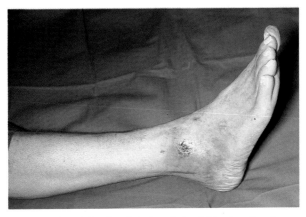

**Fig. 79** Ischaemic foot in a diabetic male. In addition to reduced or absent foot pulses, poor blood supply may be indicated by the atrophic appearance shown here with nail changes, loss of hair, slow healing and wasting.

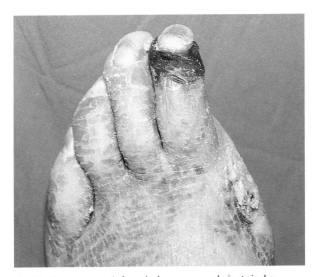

**Fig. 80** Dry gangrene. Ischaemic changes may culminate in dry gangrene with mummification of the dead tissue and a demarcation between the dead and viable tissues. The peripheral dead tissue may be painless and separate spontaneously. In this case, the first toe has been removed previously because of gangrene, which is now present distally in the second toe.

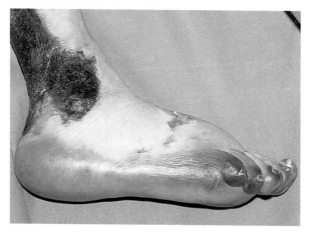

**Fig. 81** Wet gangrene. Wet gangrene is due to ischaemia with superadded infection. A foul smell suggests the presence of anaerobes which constitutes a diabetic emergency. Urgent surgery may be required in addition to optimization of glycaemic control, antibiotics and angiography.

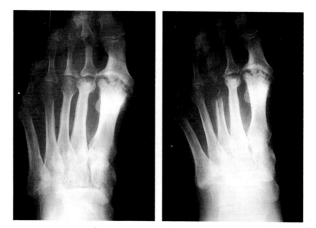

**Fig. 82** Osteomyelitis. Infection of the superficial tissues may spread to involve underlying bone. Osteomyelitis is suggested by loss of bone; dead tissue should be removed surgically. In this patient, infected neuropathic ulcers on the soles of the feet (see Fig. 125) led to osteomyelitis. These two radiographs of the left foot were taken two months apart and show the development of osteomyelitis, particularly in the third metatarsal, with rapid bone destruction.

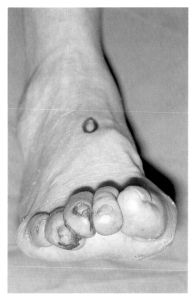

**Fig. 83** Distal microvascular disease. In some cases of peripheral ischaemia or gangrene, the peripheral pulses may be present, implying the presence of distal microvascular disease. Ulceration may also be associated with neuropathy in the presence of foot pulses. The pulses were easily palpable (dorsalis pedis pulse marked in ink) in this patient, despite the presence of painful ischaemic toes.

# LONG-TERM COMPLICATIONS: EYE DISEASE

Diabetes is now the leading cause of blindness in middle age in the Western World. As eye disease is so important, repeated screening for its early detection leading to timely treatment is mandatory. The main pathological features of the retinal microvascular changes are: capillary closure with areas of retinal non-perfusion, leaky capillaries, microaneurysms, exudates and new vessel formation (neovascularization). Retinal ischaemia is probably a major contributor to these changes. Poorly controlled diabetes itself or a change in blood glucose levels from high to low may cause transient visual blurring possibly due to osmotic shifts.

Cataracts may result from glycosylation of lens proteins. The retinal changes are broadly divided into background and proliferative. Both may initially be asymptomatic and progress to impair vision leading to blindness.

| TYPES OF EYE DISEASE |
|---|
| cataract |
| background: microaneurysms<br>dot and blot haemorrhages<br>exudates<br>maculopathy |
| transitional: intraretinal microvascular abnormalities (IRMA)<br>soft exudates<br>venous irregularity |
| proliferative: peripheral<br>disc<br>rubeosis iridis (rubeotic glaucoma) |
| retinal vein thrombosis |

**Fig. 84** Classification of diabetic eye disease.

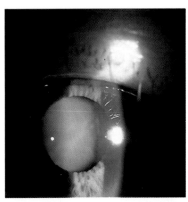

**Fig. 85** Cataract. Age-related cataract often occurs at a younger age in diabetes. The brown nuclear cataract pictured here causes gradual deterioration in vision with increasing myopia.

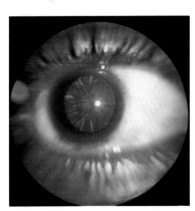

**Fig. 86** Cuneiform cataract. This type of cataract is impressive, but often causes little deterioration in vision.

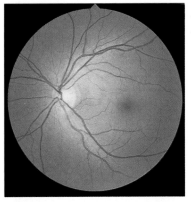

**Fig. 87** Normal fundus. The retinal vessels enter the eye at the optic disc and divide into superior and inferior, nasal (medial) and temporal (lateral) branches. The macula lies at the posterior pole of the eye and is the area with greatest visual acuity. The optic disc lies slightly nasal (medial) to the macula.

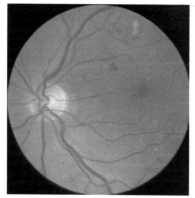

**Fig. 88**  Background retinopathy. Microaneurysms, haemorrhages and hard exudates can be seen. There is a soft exudate at 1 o'clock.

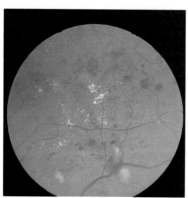

**Fig. 89**  Diabetic maculopathy. A ring of hard exudates surrounds the macula. Soft exudates, microaneurysms and deep round haemorrhages can be seen.

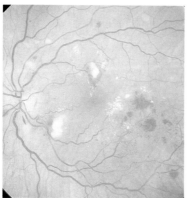

**Fig. 90**  Pre-proliferative stage of background retinopathy. This is illustrated here by large blot haemorrhages, cotton wool spots, venous irregularity and intraretinal microvascular abnormalities.

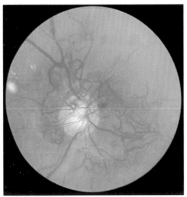

**Fig. 91** Disc new vessels. Delicate loops of new vessels grow forward towards the vitreous (note the disc haemorrhage). They carry a serious risk of blindness if untreated.

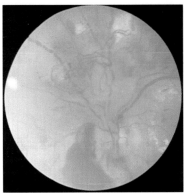

**Fig. 92** Proliferative retinopathy. Through the vitreous which is hazy from haemorrhage, can be seen proliferative and background changes. The bleeding site can be identified close to the disc and there is supero-nasal venous beading, adjacent to an area of peripheral new vessels.

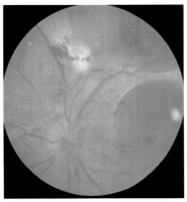

**Fig. 93** Proliferative retinopathy. This has led to an extensive traction retinal detachment.

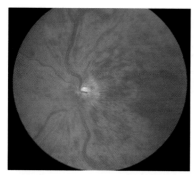

**Fig. 94** Central retinal vein occlusion. There is an increased incidence of this in diabetic patients. It presents as sudden unilateral painless loss of vision with a picture of dilated tortuous retinal veins and extensive flame-shaped intraretinal haemorrhages.

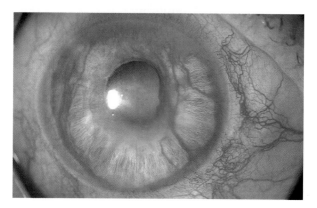

**Fig. 95** Rubeosis iridis. The ischaemia underlying diabetic proliferative retinopathy or that caused by central retinal vein occlusion may lead to new vessel formation on the iris (rubeosis iridis) resulting in a secondary glaucoma and blindness.

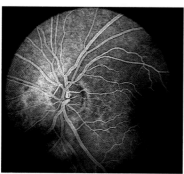

**Fig. 96** Normal fluorescein angiogram. Fluorescein angiography demonstrates the vasculature of the eye. This is a normal angiogram in the arteriovenous phase.

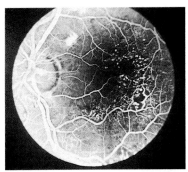

**Fig. 97** Fluorescein angiogram of severe retinopathy. There are areas of retinal non-perfusion and capillary leakage.

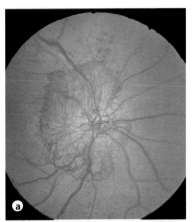

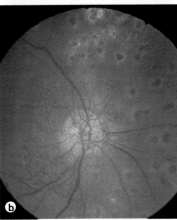

**Fig. 98** The effect of laser treatment. (a) Disc new vessels. (b) Laser photocoagulation was given and, five months later, there has been considerable resolution of the lesions.

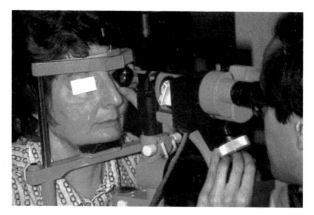

**Fig. 99**   Laser machine in use. Laser photocoagulation may halt the progression and reverse some changes of diabetic retinopathy.

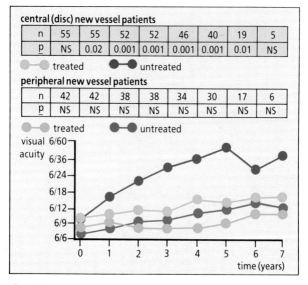

**central (disc) new vessel patients**

| n | 55 | 55 | 52 | 52 | 46 | 40 | 19 | 5 |
|---|----|----|----|----|----|----|----|---|
| p | NS | 0.02 | 0.001 | 0.001 | 0.001 | 0.001 | 0.01 | NS |

◯—◯ treated   ●—● untreated

**peripheral new vessel patients**

| n | 42 | 42 | 38 | 38 | 34 | 30 | 17 | 6 |
|---|----|----|----|----|----|----|----|---|
| p | NS | NS | NS | NS | NS | NS | NS | NS |

◯—◯ treated   ●—● untreated

**Fig. 100**   Mean visual acuity of treated and control eyes of patients with new vessels in the British Multicentre Study of photocoagulation. There was marked deterioration in eyes with disc new vessels when untreated, whilst the treated eyes deteriorated by less than one line on the Snellen chart. In patients with peripheral new vessels only, the difference between treated and untreated eyes was less, but the treated eyes still fared better.

# LONG-TERM COMPLICATIONS: RENAL TRACT

Long-duration diabetes may lead to kidney damage— nephropathy. Although many patients develop a degree of albuminuria, which is intermittent at first but constant later, not all develop the features of nephrotic syndrome: oedema, hypertension and heavy albuminuria, leading to progressive renal failure and death. Nevertheless, up to one-third of insulin-dependent patients may develop severe nephropathy which will prove fatal if untreated. The morbidity and mortality of such patients is increased by the presence of additional diabetic complications, particularly widespread vascular disease, proliferative retinopathy and severe neuropathy.

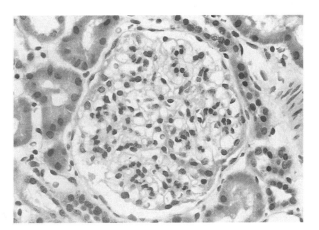

**Fig. 101** Normal glomerulus. H & E stain.

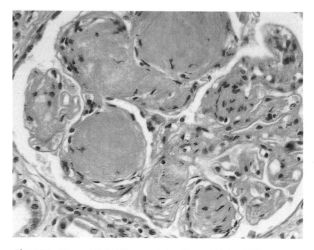

**Fig. 102** Kimmelstiel–Wilson nodules. Kimmelstiel and Wilson described patients with proteinaemia and hypertension whose glomeruli showed hyaline nodular lesions. These changes are typical of diabetic glomerulosclerosis.

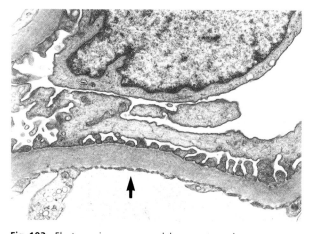

**Fig. 103** Electron microscopy reveals basement membrane thickening (arrowed) in the glomeruli of long-duration diabetic patients. This may alter the charge of the glomerular wall and affect its permeability. EM × 10,000.

| DIABETIC NEPHROPATHY | | |
|---|---|---|
| **Early phase** | **Transitional phase** | **Late phase** |
| GFR increased | GFR increased | GFR decreased |
| renal size increased | renal size increased | renal size normal or increased |
| AER increased (poor control) | AER increased (microalbuminuria) | AER greatly increased (persistent proteinuria) |
| blood pressure normal | blood pressure increased | blood pressure greatly increased |
| reversible | ?reversible | irreversible |

**Fig. 104** Natural history of diabetic nephropathy. The functional changes of diabetic nephropathy may be divided into three stages: early, transitional and late. GFR=glomerular filtration rate; AER=albumin excretion rate.

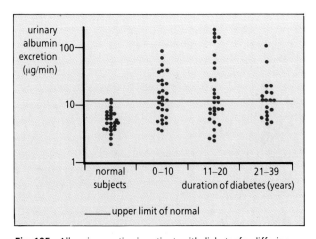

**Fig. 105** Albumin excretion in patients with diabetes for differing periods. The upper limit of normal of albumin excretion is about 30mg/24h, whereas Albustix, a reagent strip used to detect albuminuria, gives a positive reaction to urine only when the excretion rate is about 250mg/24h. The intervening rate (30–250mg/24h) is termed micro-albuminuria and it carries a risk for the development of diabetic nephropathy. Microalbuminuria may be detected by kits or radioimmunoassay.

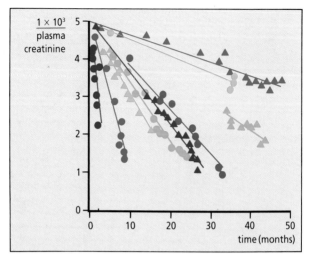

**Fig. 106** Progression of renal failure in nine diabetic patients. Once albuminuria has become established, renal deterioration proceeds inexorably. The rate of decline may be documented by plotting the inverse of the plasma creatinine level. Different patients have different rates of decline. The only factor that is known to slow this decline is the aggressive treatment of hypertension. Improving glycaemic control may reduce the microalbumin excretion rate, but probably has little or no effect on established nephropathy.

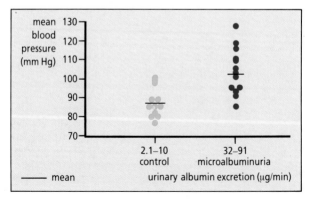

**Fig. 107** Blood pressure in diabetic patients with or without microalbuminuria. Hypertension is associated with the development of nephropathy and its aggressive treatment may slow the progression of renal impairment.

| ADVANCED DIABETIC NEPHROPATHY | |
|---|---|
| **Treatment** | **Problems** |
| haemodialysis | vascular access<br>haemodynamic instability<br>progression of retinopathy |
| continuous ambulatory peritoneal dialysis (CAPD) | peritoneal infection<br>glucose loads in peritoneal dialysis fluid<br>continuous attention required |
| transplantation | availability of kidneys<br>immunosuppression<br>nephropathy in graft |

**Fig. 108** Treatment options for advanced diabetic nephropathy and their problems.

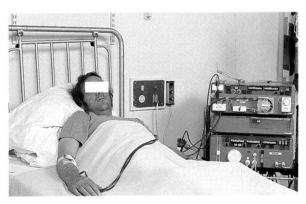

**Fig. 109** Patient undergoing haemodialysis.

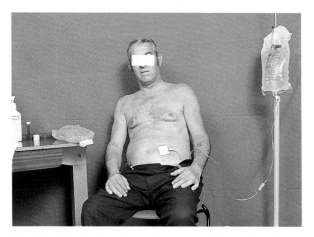

**Fig. 110** Patient undergoing continuous ambulatory peritoneal dialysis.

# LONG-TERM COMPLICATIONS: THE NEUROPATHIES

## DIABETIC NEUROPATHIES

peripheral motor

peripheral sensory

peripheral mixed motor and sensory

isolated cranial nerve palsies

mononeuritis

diabetic amyotrophy

autonomic neuropathy

**Fig. 111** Diabetic neuropathy. Diabetes causes a wide variety of disturbances in the nervous system. The mechanisms by which they are caused may include contributions from microvascular damage and altered neural metabolism.

## AETIOLOGY OF DIABETIC NEUROPATHY

demyelination

axon loss

infarction

blocked vessels (ischaemia)

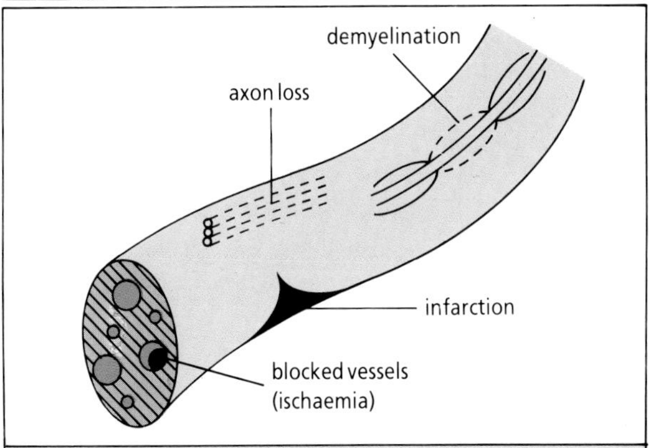

nerve metabolism:   glucose ↑
sorbitol ↓ ↑
myo-inositol ↓

**Fig. 112** Aetiology of diabetic neuropathy. Metabolic and vascular changes may both contribute to the aetiology.

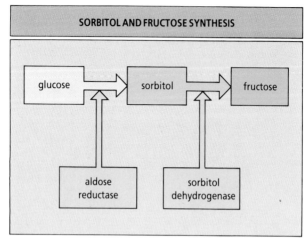

**SORBITOL AND FRUCTOSE SYNTHESIS**

glucose → sorbitol → fructose

aldose reductase

sorbitol dehydrogenase

**Fig. 113** Conversion of glucose to fructose via sorbitol. Fructose and sorbitol accumulate in the peripheral nerves of diabetic patients. It has been suggested, but not proven, that their presence in excess is partly responsible for human diabetic neuropathy. Drugs which inhibit aldose reductase are under investigation as possible treatments for the prevention or reversal of neuropathy.

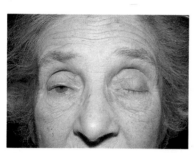

**Fig. 114** Complete third cranial nerve palsy. A third nerve lesion is the commonest cranial nerve lesion seen in diabetes.

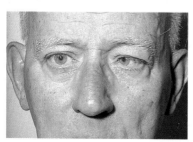

**Fig. 115** Right sixth cranial nerve lesion. Diplopia occurs upon looking to the right.

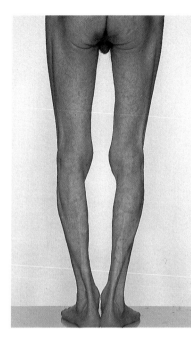

**Fig. 116** Generalized wasting of the muscles. This may produce a proximal or peripheral weakness, or both. Diabetic cachexia is associated with autonomic neuropathy, particularly diarrhoea.

| PERIPHERAL NEUROPATHY |
| --- |
| **Symptoms** |
| paraesthesiae ('pins and needles')<br>numbness<br>lack of pain sensation (injuries unnoticed)<br>dysthesiae (abnormal sensations), e.g. 'walking on cotton wool'<br>hyperaesthesiae, e.g. bedclothes cause painful sensations in legs |
| **Signs** |
| tendon reflexes: diminished or absent<br>sensation: diminished or absent<br>muscle wasting<br>deformity, e.g. dropped metatarsal heads<br>ulcers |

**Fig. 117** Features of peripheral neuropathy.

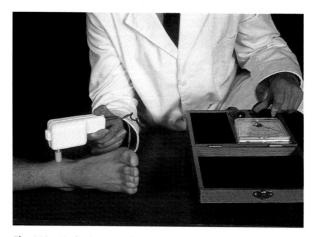

**Fig. 118** Biothesiometer. This instrument enables measurement of vibration perception threshold.

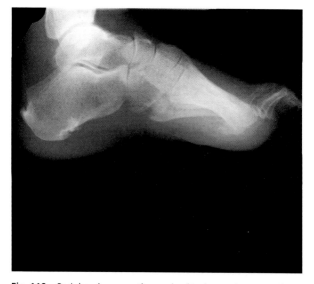

**Fig. 119** Peripheral neuropathy may lead to dropped metatarsal heads producing a degree of pes cavus which, in turn, predisposes to ulceration. This lateral radiograph shows an accentuated arch with dropped metatarsal heads; the first toe has been amputated previously because of gangrene. There is a calcaneal spur, a common finding in diabetes.

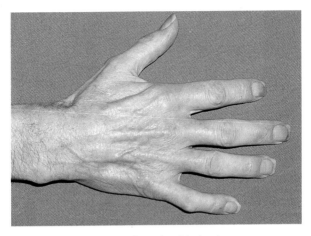

**Fig. 120**  Wasting of the small muscles of the hand.

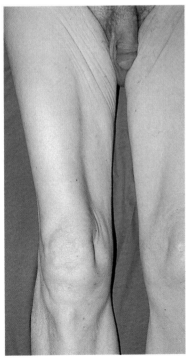

**Fig. 121**  Wasting of the thigh muscles, especially affecting the right adductor group and quadriceps femoris in a patient with marked neuropathy.

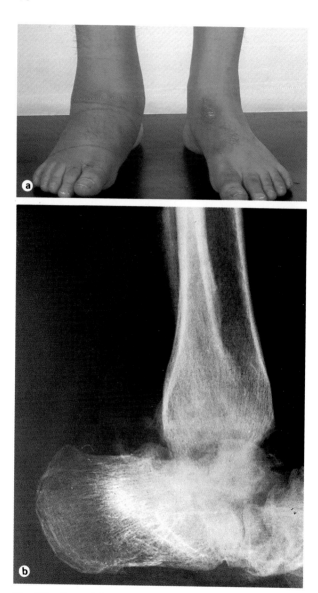

**Fig. 122** Charcot joint. As it produces a severe peripheral neuropathy, diabetes is one of the causes of neuropathic joint disorganization, the 'Charcot' joint. This patient has disorganized ankle and subtalar joints. (a) Clinical and (b) radiographic appearances.

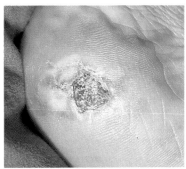

**Fig. 123** Foot ulcer. Lack of normal sensation in the foot predisposes to injury and ulceration. This patient accidentally dropped a walnut shell into her slipper and walked on it for several days without noticing. The resultant ulcer was painless. Ill-fitting footwear is a major cause of ulceration.

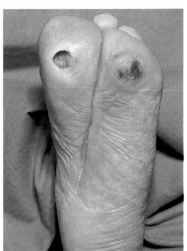

**Fig. 124** Foot ulcer. Neuropathic ulcers may become chronic and, despite healing after prolonged rest, may quickly relapse. This patient has chronic painless ulcers which have been present bilaterally for many years. Several toes and a wedge of foot have been resected previously.

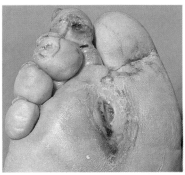

**Fig. 125** Foot ulcer. This patient has easily controlled NIDDM, but peripheral neuropathy complicated by infected painless ulcers on the soles of the feet. The toes and web spaces are infected with *Staphylococcus aureus* and there is underlying osteomyelitis (see also Fig. 82).

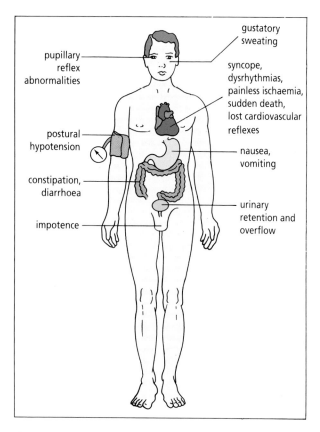

**Fig. 126** Some features of autonomic neuropathy.

| TESTS FOR AUTONOMIC NEUROPATHY |
| --- |
| heart rate response to: standing |
| deep breathing |
| Valsalva manoeuvre |
| blood pressure response to: standing |
| hand-grip |
| pupil size response to light |

**Fig. 127** Some tests used to detect for the presence of autonomic neuropathy.

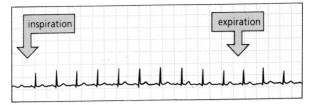

**Fig. 128** ECG in autonomic neuropathy. In the normal subject, deep breathing accentuates the normal sinus arrhythmia. In autonomic neuropathy, this response is lost. During the test, the subject breathes slowly and deeply (six breaths per minute), while the ECG continuously records a rhythm strip. Usually the heart rate difference between inspiration (rate increases) and expiration (rate decreases) is at least ten beats per minute. In the presence of autonomic neuropathy, this response is lost and the rate varies little as shown here.

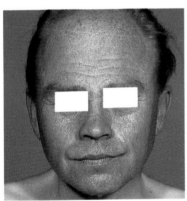

**Fig. 129** Facial flushing and sweating after eating in a patient with autonomic neuropathy. Gustatory sweating (after tasting food) is a helpful symptom indicating autonomic neuropathy and it may be induced by particular foods, such as cheese.

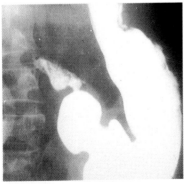

**Fig. 130** Barium meal showing a distended stomach due to stasis from autonomic gastroparesis. The barium was taken two hours before this radiograph.

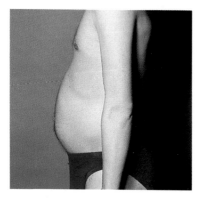

**Fig. 131** Distended bladder due to autonomic neuropathy. This young male presented with painless swelling of the lower abdomen. He was not impotent, indicating the highly selective damage which can occur in autonomic disease.

---

### DIABETIC IMPOTENCE

prevalence: common; up to one-third diabetic men

symptoms: libido usually preserved
absence of morning erections
absence of erections with full bladder

signs: other features of autonomic or peripheral neuropathy
peripheral vascular disease

investigations: endocrinology normal

**Fig. 132** Features of diabetic impotence.

---

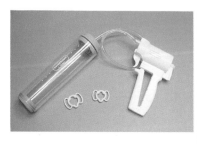

**Fig. 133** Erecaid. This is a vacuum-forming device which helps to produce an erection in patients with impotence. The erection is maintained by an elastic band around the base of the penis. Alternatively, a surgical prosthesis may be implanted or the patient may inject his penis with papaverine to produce an erection.

# DIABETES AND THE SKIN

Patients with diabetes may develop a wide range of skin, soft tissue and joint conditions. These may be due to the propensity of diabetic patients to develop infectious, vasculitic changes in the skin and, possibly, due to glycosylation of structural proteins.

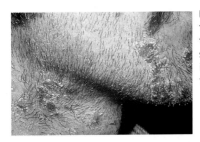

**Fig. 134** Staphylococcal folliculitis occurring on the beard area. When several follicles are involved, the lesion is termed a carbuncle.

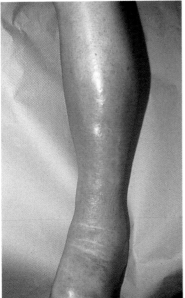

**Fig. 135** Streptococcal cellulitis. This is a very common skin complication of diabetes. It usually results from a minor crack in the skin or injury which acts as a portal of entry for infection. The hot, painful, shiny red lesion spreads proximally and may cause local lymphadenopathy, systemic upset and poor glycaemic control.

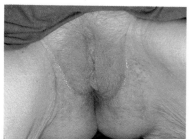

**Fig. 136** Candidal vulvitis. This is a common way for diabetes to present to the dermatologist, venereologist or gynaecologist.

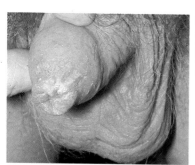

**Fig. 137** *Candida albicans.* Infection of the glans and prepuce may be a presenting complication of NIDDM.

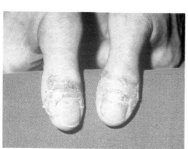

**Fig. 138** Chronic candidal paronychia. There is loss of the nail cuticle and ridging of the nail secondary to the inflammation of the nail fold.

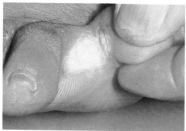

**Fig. 139** Dermatophytosis: tinea pedis. This fungal infection commonly starts in the forth toe web and then spreads on to the dorsum of the foot and into the nails.

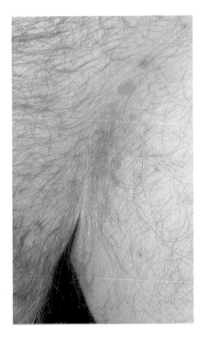

**Fig. 140** Intertrigo of the groin due to *Candida albicans*.

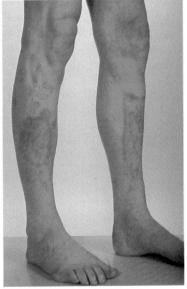

**Fig. 141** Necrobiosis lipoidica diabeticorum. The plaques on the front of both shins are characteristic.

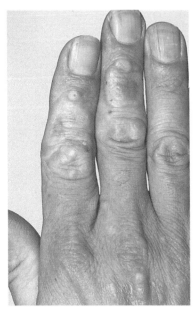

**Fig. 142** Granuloma annulare. The lesions are seen as flesh-coloured, slightly shiny, rings and nodules on the fingers.

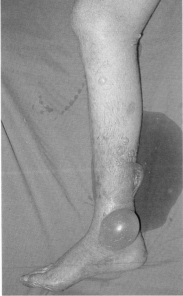

**Fig. 143** Idiopathic diabetic bullae. These arise at the epidermal–dermal junction.

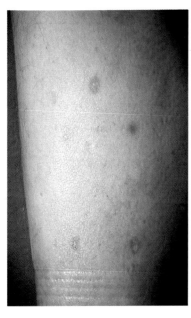

**Fig. 144** Diabetic dermopathy. The usual distribution on the lower legs is shown. These lesions result in small atrophic, shiny, white scars.

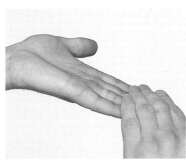

**Fig. 145** Diabetic cheiroarthropathy. Changes in the soft tissues and joints of the hands may cause stiffness. At an early stage, there is an inability to hyperextend the metacarpophalangeal joints, which this patient is attempting to do.

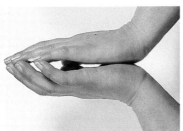

**Fig. 146** Diabetic cheiroarthropathy. At a later stage than that shown in Fig. 145, the patient has limited joint mobility and some clawing.

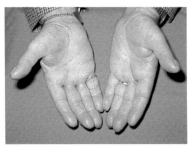

**Fig. 147** Chronic diabetic hands. Lundbaek described the changes that occur in the hands of patients with diabetes of long duration. They are stiff, slightly swollen and reminiscent of systemic sclerosis.

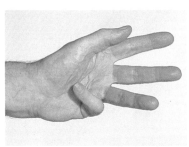

**Fig. 148** Dupuytren's contracture. There is thickening and contraction of the palmar fascia. This may be associated with the presence of diabetes.

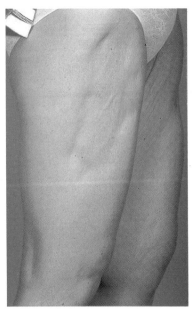

**Fig. 149** Lipoatrophy. Loss of subcutaneous fat may occur at the site of insulin injections. Its basis may be immunological and with the change to less immunogenic insulins, these lesions should become rare.

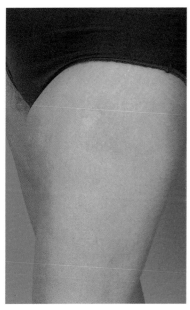

**Fig. 150** Lipo-hypertrophy. Repeated insulin injections at the same site may lead to a local increase in subcutaneous fat.

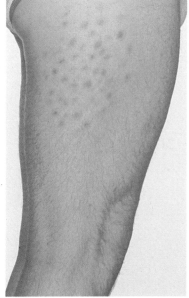

**Fig. 151** Intracutaneous injections. Insulin is injected subcutaneously, but if injected erroneously into the skin produces the lesions shown here.

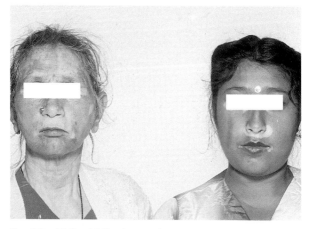

**Fig. 152** Vitiligo. Vitiligo is pure white as opposed to the hypopigmented changes seen in diseases such as leprosy. It is associated with a wide range of autoimmune endocrine conditions, including diabetes, and is often familial. The mother (left) and daughter illustrated here, both have vitiligo; the former has thyrotoxicosis and the latter no endocrine condition at present.

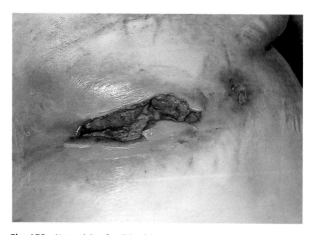

**Fig. 153** Necrotizing fasciitis. This acute necrotic process affecting the subcutaneous tissues is associated with diabetes. It is due to infection with mixed organisms, including anaerobes. It may prove rapidly fatal unless treated urgently with surgery and antibiotics. This middle-aged woman with NIDDM developed necrotizing fasciitis of the right upper quadrant of the abdomen, which proved fatal.

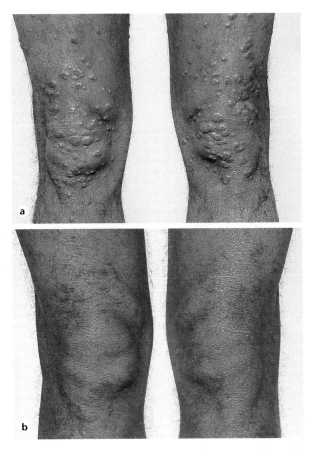

**Fig. 154** Eruptive xanthomata in a 35-year-old Asian man with poorly controlled NIDDM. The lesions (a) were much improved after two years of insulin treatment (b).

# DIABETES IN CHILDREN

The incidence of IDDM in children is thought to be increasing, making it one of the more common chronic diseases of childhood. Its current prevalence in the UK is approximately two per thousand children by sixteen years of age.

| PRESENTING FEATURES OF CHILDHOOD DIABETES |
|---|
| polyuria |
| nocturia |
| thirst |
| enuresis |
| weight loss |
| poor growth |
| lassitude |
| increased appetite |
| monilial infection |
| ketoacidosis |

**Fig. 155** Presenting features of diabetes in children.

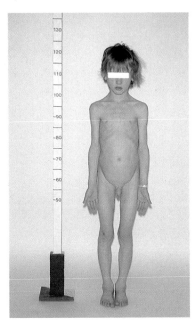

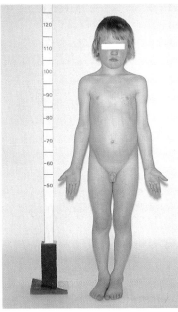

**Fig. 156** Before and after insulin treatment. This child illustrates the weight loss and subsequent weight gain just two months after the introduction of insulin treatment.

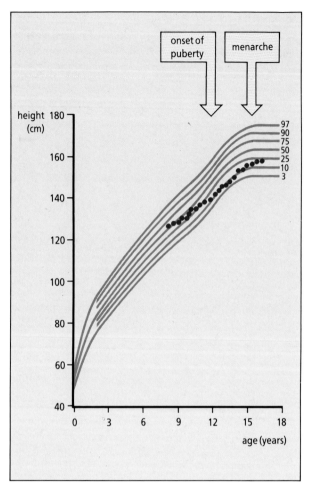

**Fig. 157** Centile growth chart 1: height. Progress of growth in diabetic children should be carefully monitored by regularly plotting height and weight on centile charts. Periods of poor diabetic control may be associated with slowing of growth and poor weight gain, while obesity, associated with excessive insulin dosage (over-insulinization) or over-eating is not uncommon. This centile chart is from a girl who developed diabetes at the age of eight years. Although on the 50th centile for height initially, she followed the 10th centile for a time and was near the 25th centile at age sixteen years. The onset of puberty at age 11.5 years was slightly delayed, while menarche at age 15.5 years was quite delayed.

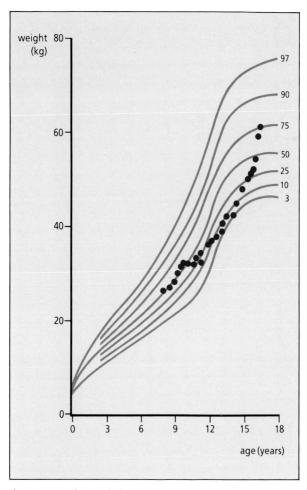

**Fig. 158** Centile growth chart 2: weight. This chart is that of the same girl as in Fig. 157. Her weight, like her height, was also on the 50th centile at diagnosis, was relatively low in early teenage years, but was high in later teenage years. Such a case illustrates that childhood and adolescent diabetes is often a difficult condition to treat.

### INSULIN TREATMENT IN CHILDREN

once-daily injection often sufficient before puberty

twice-daily injections usually required during and after puberty

insulin dosage guide: 0.5 – 1.0 u/kg/day

psychological disturbance may hamper management during teenage years

**Fig. 159** Particular points regarding insulin treatment in children.

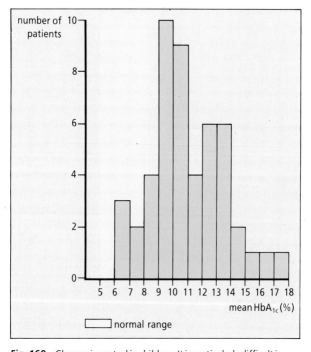

**Fig. 160** Glycaemic control in children. It is particularly difficult in children to achieve normoglycaemia throughout the daily cycle. This bar chart shows that the majority of 49 children attending a clinic did not have a normal $HbA_{1c}$ value (means of the twelve-month values are plotted; overall mean value of all measurements was 10.9%). Control of diabetes is better during the first one or two years after diagnosis, when there is likely to be residual insulin secretion.

# DIABETES, PREGNANCY AND CONTRACEPTION

The prognosis for pregnancy in the diabetic patient has improved considerably. Twenty years ago, the fetal loss rate was up to 25%. Today, in specialist centres, it is only 4–5% and may be approaching that in non-diabetic women. This improvement results largely from the intensive management of diabetes throughout pregnancy and allowing delivery to be as near to term as possible.

| PREGNANCY AND DIABETES |
|---|
| ketosis more likely in diabetic mothers |
| possible worsening of diabetic complications, e.g. retinopathy |
| pre-eclampsia and hydramnios more common |
| malformations three times as common in infants or diabetic mothers |
| macrosomia may cause difficulties at delivery |
| further fetal problems may be produced by planned premature delivery |
| perinatal mortality exceeds normal |
| perinatal morbidity exceeds normal |

**Fig. 161** Potential problems of pregnancy in the diabetic patient.

| POTENTIAL PROBLEMS OF INFANT |
|---|
| congenital malformations |
| macrosomia (large, obese baby) |
| fetal distress |
| jaundice |
| hypoglycaemic seizures |
| respiratory distress syndrome |

**Fig. 162** Potential problems of the infant of a diabetic mother.

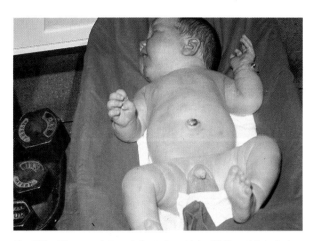

**Fig. 163** Macrosomia in an infant who weighed 5.6kg at birth. Such an appearance and weight suggest uncontrolled diabetes during pregnancy.

## FACTORS INDICATING GDM

| | |
|---|---|
| gestational diabetes in a previous pregnancy | previous malformed infant |
| family history of diabetes | maternal obesity |
| previously large babies | development of hydramnios |
| previous unexplained fetal death | development of macrosomia |
| | glycosuria |

**Fig. 164** Gestational diabetes. In addition to pregnancy in an established diabetic patient, diabetes may appear during pregnancy. This is termed 'gestational diabetes mellitus' (GDM). GDM may be suspected for one or more of the reasons shown here. Repeated oral glucose tolerance testing (OGTT) during pregnancy may show the development of GDM. The lowered renal threshold for glucose in pregnancy makes glycosuria common and does not allow the diagnosis of diabetes without an OGTT. Borderline cases are termed 'impaired glucose tolerance' and also require careful supervision of blood glucose levels throughout pregnancy.

## MANAGEMENT OF DIABETES IN PREGNANCY

1. Aim to achieve normoglycaemia throughout 24h period (ideally blood glucose always < 6.5mmol/l; $HbA_{1c}$ in normal range).
2. Patients monitor blood glucose levels at home using test strips (before and after meals; up to 7 tests daily).
3. Oral hypoglycaemic agents not advised.
4. Try diet alone in cases of NIDDM, GDM and gestational IGT; if control unsatisfactory, transfer to insulin.
5. Give insulin by 1–4 injections daily or use CSII to maintain normoglycaemia.
6. Review frequently throughout pregnancy at a joint diabetes/ antenatal clinic.
7. Prepregnancy counselling: optimizing glycaemic control before conception and in first trimester may reduce congenital malformations.

**Fig. 165** Principles of management of diabetes in pregnancy.

## MANAGEMENT OF PREGNANCY AND LABOUR

1. Deliver as near term as possible.

2. Deliver in hospital.

3. Assess stage of pregnancy using ultrasound and lecithin/sphingomyelin ratio.

4. If insulin treated, during labour:
   (i) infuse 5% or 10% dextrose i.v., each litre 8-hourly;
   (ii) infuse soluble insulin i.v. by infusion pump or add to i.v. dextrose solution;
   (iii) insulin usually stopped after delivery in NIDDM, GDM and gestational IGT cases;
   (iv) resume previous insulin regimen in IDDM cases;
   (v) insulin requirements may be increased while breast-feeding.

**Fig. 166** Principles of management of pregnancy and labour.

## CONTRACEPTION AND DIABETES

preferred methods:

barrier methods: condom or cap

intrauterine contraceptive device (IUCD)

progestagen only pill

'safe' period

**Fig. 167** Contraception. The combined oestrogen/progestagen pill is not advised because of the potential, although small, increased risk of vascular complications in the diabetic patient. Monilial infection may be a problem in diabetic women who take the pill.

# DIABETES AND SURGERY

The management of diabetes during surgery presents a common problem in hospital practice. Uncontrolled diabetes may lead to increased morbidity and mortality. For the purpose of outlining management plans, diabetic patients may be classified as: (i) NIDDM (diet treatment only); (ii) NIDDM (diet and tablet treatment); and (iii) IDDM (insulin treatment). Operations may be classified as: (i) minor (e.g. hernia repair or appendicectomy); and (ii) major (e.g. bowel resection, cholecystectomy or coronary artery bypass).

---

### MANAGEMENT OF THE DIABETIC SURGICAL PATIENT

1. Admit to hospital all known diabetic patients 24 – 48h prior to elective surgery.
2. Stop oral hypoglycaemic agents 24h before surgery.
3. Aim to control diabetes; ideally blood glucose level 4 – 8 mmol/l.
4. Aim to prevent catabolism.
5. Try not to starve patient for too long.

**Fig. 168** Principles of management of the diabetic surgical patient.

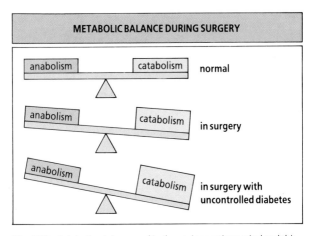

**Fig. 169** Catabolism is increased in the perioperative period and this is dramatically increased if diabetes is present and uncontrolled.

### MANAGEMENT OF NIDDM: DIET ONLY TREATMENT

1. Fasting is not usually a problem.

2. Check random blood glucose (RBG) before, during and after operation.

3. If RBG satisfactory:
   minor operation, no additional treatment;
   major operation, no additional treatment.

4. If RBG high, consider insulin (subcutaneous or i.v. infusion).

**Fig. 170**  Management plan A: NIDDM, diet only treatment.

### MANAGEMENT OF NIDDM DIET AND TABLET TREATMENT

1. Stop oral hypoglycaemic agents at least 24h before elective surgery.

2. Fasting is not usually a problem.

3. Check RBG before, during and after operation.

4. If RBG satisfactory:
   minor operation, no additional treatment;
   major operation, no additional treatment.

5. If RBG high, consider insulin (subcutaneous or i.v. infusion).

**Fig. 171**  Management plan B: NIDDM, diet and tablet treatment.

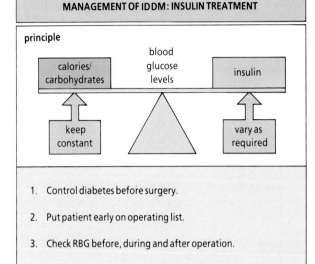

**MANAGEMENT OF IDDM: INSULIN TREATMENT**

principle

| calories/carbohydrates | blood glucose levels | insulin |

keep constant — vary as required

1. Control diabetes before surgery.

2. Put patient early on operating list.

3. Check RBG before, during and after operation.

4. Insulin: omit usual morning subcutaneous dose; change to i.v. soluble insulin given by infusion pump or added to drip fluid (rate, e.g. 1–3u/h).

5. i.v. fluids: 5% or 10% dextrose;
   each litre 8-hourly (i.e. 600kcals/24h);
   add 20–40 mmol/l KCl.

6. Eating: when resumed, restart usual subcutaneous insulin;
   if delayed, give insulin i.v. or subcutaneously and consider i.v. feeding.

**Fig. 172** Management plan C: IDDM, insulin treatment.

# THE DIABETIC CLINIC

Diabetic patients may be reviewed in hospital clinics, by their general practitioner, by both (shared care) or by no-one. Some traditional hospital diabetic clinics have been replaced by purpose-built diabetes centres. They offer daily outpatient attendances and provide treatment with an emphasis on patient education.

| PURPOSES OF DIABETIC CLINIC |
|---|
| 1. Provide patient education. |
| 2. Prevent and screen for diabetic complications. |
| 3. Treat established complications. |
| 4. Optimize blood glucose control. |

**Fig. 173** Purposes of the diabetic clinic.

| MONITORING DIABETES |
|---|
| **Measurements made at diabetic clinic** |
| weight |
| height |
| centile charts (children) |
| urine: glucose, ketones, albumin and microalbuminuria |
| blood glucose level, $HbA_{1c}$% and fructosamine |
| blood pressure |
| **Measurements made at home** |
| blood glucose levels |
| urine: glucose and ketones |

**Fig. 174** Measurements made at the diabetic clinic and at home by patients to monitor the control of their condition.

## SCREENING FOR DIABETIC COMPLICATIONS

take history of symptoms and check for physical signs:

| | |
|---|---|
| eye disease: | visual acuity |
| | fundoscopy |
| | intraocular pressure |
| | fluorescein angiography |
| renal disease: | albuminuria and 24h protein excretion |
| | blood pressure |
| | plasma creatinine |
| foot disease: | inspection and clinical examination |
| | (blood and nerve supply) |
| | Doppler ultrasound blood flow |
| | nerve conduction studies |
| cardiac disease: | chest radiography |
| | ECG |
| referrals to specialist clinics: | ophthalmic, renal, vascular and orthopaedic |

**Fig. 175** Screening for diabetic complications.

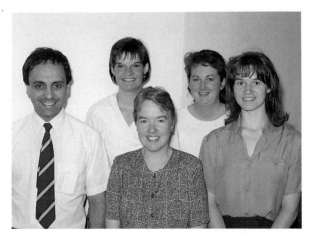

**Fig. 176** Members of the health care team. This includes doctors, dietitians, specialist diabetes liaison nurses/health visitors, chiropodist and clinic nurses.

**REASONS FOR FAULTY COMPLIANCE WITH TREATMENT**

patient does not understand treatment or reasons for it

treatment perceived as too arduous

patient has difficulty appreciating long-term benefit of treatment

**Fig. 177** Compliance with treatment. It is easy with experience to prescribe treatment for diabetes. For the patient, however, lifelong adherence to a diet, a regimen of daily injections or tablets and home monitoring of urine or blood glucose is initially bewildering and then arduous. Not surprisingly, many patients fail to comply with what they perceive as a tedious set of instructions and some default from clinic attendance.

**REASONS FOR DEFAULT FROM CLINIC**

patients have to wait too long

patients see different doctor each visit

junior doctors have little experience of diabetes

consultation time is short; doctor and clinic look busy

different doctors give conflicting advice

patient considers nothing worthwhile happens at clinic

doctor–patient conflict

**Fig. 178** Possible reasons for default from clinic.

# INDEX

# NOTES

# NOTES

# NOTES